GOODBYE, DRY EYE!

EXPERT ADVICE ON REMEDIES
AND RELIEF FOR DRY EYES

SHILPI PRADHAN, MD
BOARD CERTIFIED OPHTHALMOLOGIST
DRY EYE SPECIALIST

Disclaimer Notice:

This book is intended for education only. This book is not intended to be a substitute for the medical advice of a licensed physician. The readers should consult with their doctor in any matters relating to their health. This book contains information intended to help readers be better-informed healthcare consumers. It is presented as general advice on healthcare. Always consult your doctor for your individual needs. Please consult your local eye doctor or an ophthalmologist to know what medical or surgical treatments are right for you. All medical care should be individualized to you and your unique situation. All opinions presented are that of Dr. Shilpi Pradhan.

Cover image used with free standard license by Jonathan Borba:

https://www.pexels.com/photo/brown-human-eye-2873058/.

To my husband (Dr. Kumar Abhishek), my children (Shreya, Ankit, Asha, and Priya), my parents (Dr. Shekhar Pradhan and Savita Pradhan), and my siblings and their families, who are all my constant supporters. I love you all. Thank you for your support.

"Learn from yesterday, live for today, hope for tomorrow. The important thing is not to stop questioning."
– Albert Einstein

CONTENTS

TESTIMONIALS ON WHY YOU SHOULD READ THIS BOOK!

"Dr. Pradhan has written a comprehensive book on dry eye in language that is easily understood by patients. She explains the most commonly asked questions in a dry eye practice: Do I have watery eyes because my eyes are dry? It is not doctor-speak. A must-read!" – Dr. Mitra Ayazifar, MD, Capital Eye Medical Group.

"Dr. Pradhan has created the ideal, comprehensive guide for Dry Eye and MGD patients to better understand their conditions and the treatment recommendations. A more knowledgeable patient is a more successful one!" – Dr. Laura Periman, MD, Dry Eye Master, Periman Eye Institute, Seattle, WA.

"Dr. Pradhan does a deep dive into the all-too-prevalent and debilitating disease of dry eye – often being undertreated in so many patients! She explains the symptoms, anatomy, contributing factors, and nuances of the disease in an accessible manner. Her book is full of valuable educational information written in a conversational tone. She provides patients with the knowledge to understand the disease, be proactive about treatment, and take back their lives!" – Dr. Deborah Wu, MD, Shoreline Vision, MI.

Goodbye, Dry Eye! is a much-needed, comprehensive text that provides the answers to all of your nagging dry eye questions and more. The conversation-style format allows Dr. Pradhan to communicate with the reader in relatable terms at a level that any layperson could understand and with enough depth and specificity that taught even a seasoned comprehensive ophthalmologist a lot. A must-read, especially for people that have already "tried it all." – Dr. Patricia Nelson, MD, FACS, Minnesota Eye Institute.

"A comprehensive book to learn all about your dry eyes. This book walks you through the causes and, most importantly, helps you understand what to expect and how your physician will guide and treat you through the options available with up-to-date treatment plans." – Dr. Shruthi Chandrashekhar MD, DiplABOM, Dipl ABLM, Zoestyle Medicine, Glen Allen, VA.

"This is a must-read for any patient suffering from dry eyes. Dr. Pradhan breaks down dry eyes in a way that patients can understand to help them understand their disease and get relief. As a physician who treats many dry eye patients, I plan to recommend this to my patients as well!" – Dr. Keshini Parbhu, MD, Ophthalmology, Oculofacial Surgery, Remagin, Windermere, FL.

For patient testimonials, please check out **our Google reviews** by searching reviews for Eye Doctor MD PC as well as for Dr. Shilpi Pradhan and also on her website.

INTRODUCTION

Welcome to your pocket-sized guide to dry eye disease by me, Dr. Shilpi Pradhan, a board-certified ophthalmologist, and dry eye specialist. I became a dry eye specialist out of need as I myself have dry eyes, and so many people have untreated dry eyes and are miserable. Other doctors refer patients to me every week who have just been given samples of artificial tears and are told to figure out which one works the best. There is a systematic way to evaluate and treat dry eyes. Sometimes you may not "feel" any difference (just like you don't feel different when you treat your high blood pressure with medication), but dry eye medications and specific treatments do help dry eyes, depending on the cause of your dry eyes.

Dry eye disease (DED), also known as dysfunctional tear syndrome, is a chronic condition. It has a prevalence of about 15% in the U.S. population, but it is more common in women and people as we get older (over 60 years old) (Rege et al.). There is no cure for it, but there are many effective treatments for it. We are going to go through dry eye disease in a brief but systematic way. The material is presented in a way that you can easily understand even if you don't have a medical background. If we can determine what is wrong, we can treat it more effectively. My hope for you is to get some answers and solutions from this book and some questions to ask your eye doctor to help you get the relief you need. Please consult your local eye doctor or ophthalmologist to know what medical or surgical treatments are right for you. All medical care should be individualized to you and your unique situation.

We will talk about the basics of dry eye disease, including learning some eye and eyelid anatomy, the normal tear film, and the major causes of dry eye disease. This is not a comprehensive scientific review. It is a guide to help you get the relief you need and learn about what doctors take into account with a "simple" dry eye exam. You will see why I can't do a dry eye exam at the same time as your regular exam. Dry eye is a real disease, and it has been extensively studied, especially with the Tear Film and Ocular Surface Society Dry Eye WorkShop (TFOS DEWS) studies published in 2007 and again in 2017 with updated recommendations.

The tear film is made up of two layers: the oil layer, which protects your water layer from evaporating, and the water layer, which has the nutrients and mucin your eye needs to keep nourished and healthy. You need both layers and all components of the tear film to be of <u>normal quality and quantity</u> to not have dry eyes. We sometimes talk about these two layers as separate disease processes, sometimes coined as "aqueous deficiency" (or missing the water layer) or "evaporative" (missing the oil layer so the water layer evaporates faster), but truly speaking, most people have a mixture of both types. Most of us have some degree of dry eye these days with our constant computer use. We're learning more and more about how inflammation is possibly the root cause of dry eye disease in all the layers of the ocular surface. Controlling that ocular surface and systemic (whole body) inflammation can be the key to controlling your dry eye disease as well as keeping the dry eye cycle functioning properly with the corneal nerve feedback loop. We will also get into normal eye anatomy with some diagrams later in the book.

You may be wondering why you should bother treating dry eyes anyway if you can see well most of the time. It has been studied that there is a substantial economic burden from dry eye disease from decreased productivity in the workplace as well as psychological effects from the pain a patient may suffer from dry eye disease. Ignoring dry eye can also lead to corneal changes such as Salzmann's or corneal ulcers, which may need surgical intervention later. It is not a problem that can go away on its own. We need you to take charge of your health, and we (your doctors and I) are here to help. That's why I'm writing this book. Let's get started and hope something in this book resonates with you and enables you to improve your eye health!

1

COMMON SYMPTOMS

"DOC, MY EYE BURNS AND FEELS DRY."

"DOC, MY EYE FEELS SANDY/GRITTY."

"DOC, I CAN'T SEE."

W hen my patients come in with specific symptoms, I know they have dry eye disease. The most common symptom is a complaint of eye pain and dryness. Other symptoms that may not be as obvious include feeling like something is in their eyes, a sandy or gritty sensation, watering, and pain when opening their eyes in the morning, or even painful eyes all day long. A common confusing symptom is blurry vision that comes and goes. Sometimes patients wonder if they have cataracts or macular degeneration, or glaucoma with intermittent blurry vision, and I explain to them that those conditions do not come and go. Either they are present and causing their blurry vision, or they are not. Whereas in dry eye disease, the tear film or ocular surface keeps changing as the tears and environment change and then your vision changes. It is like the windshield wiper of your car. When it is clear with blinks or wipes, then your vision is clear, but when the surface is irregular (with rain on the windshield, for example), your vision can be blurry. I ask, "**Can you blink it away?**" and if the answer is yes, then the cause of the blurry vision is dry eye disease.

There are a few other diseases like Fuchs' dystrophy, which is a hereditary corneal disease, which can cause fluctuating vision, usually worse in the mornings or after a nap. Anyone who has had radial keratotomy (RK) surgery can also have fluctuating vision depending on the time of day and intraocular pressure changes resulting in up to 0.5 diopters of change in your glasses prescription too. If this sounds like you, talk to your eye doctor about it.

"DOC, MY EYELASHES ARE CRUSTY."

You may notice that you have crusty eyelashes, called blepharitis, especially in the morning. You may wake up with "sleep" in the corner of your eyes. This can be from a number of causes, including sleeping with your eyes open or an eyelid infection from skin bacteria, or even a mite called Demodex folliculorum that loves to live in eyelashes and skin follicles. This mite is a common cause of dry eye disease and fluctuating vision in my patients. It is also associated with facial rosacea. In fact, one of the FDA-approved treatments for rosacea is ivermectin 1% cream, an anti-parasite cream to kill Demodex. It also helps facial rosacea in the process. I don't always treat Demodex if the patient does not want to treat themselves and the mites are not causing a problem. I do recommend daily hygiene to prevent the mites from proliferating significantly and keeping your eyelashes clean which can help your vision and dry eye disease.

"DOC, MY EYES JUST HURT."

Painful dry eye disease is a specific subgroup we will discuss later, but it has been called "neuropathic dry eye." It can occur with chronic untreated dry eyes to the point where patients may have to sit with their eyes closed in a dark room all the time. It has been shown on confocal microscopy (a complex way to look at the corneal cells in a living person) that your corneal nerves can become damaged and have small knots on the ends of the corneal nerves called neuromas. These abnormal neuromas can send pain signals even when the dry eye is improved on your clinical exam. You may think about this like post-shingles pain (also called post-herpetic neuralgia) which can be felt in the area of shingles involvement. When shingles pain occurs around the eye, it is called trigeminal neuralgia, as the shingles virus often affects the trigeminal nerve or the nerve that provides feeling to the face and parts of the neck.

Corneal surface (epithelium) damage can cause corneal nerve damage, which can cause abnormal feedback loops and worsen dry eye disease. The abnormal feedback loops can actually go both ways as well—patients can have too much sensation or abnormal pain, or they can have too little sensation and develop dry eye that they cannot feel. This lack of feeling can also be a problem because patients can come back with severe corneal ulcers or melts from a lack of corneal healing and not even know it. We call this "neurotrophic keratitis," where patients cannot even feel the corneal damage they have.

I had a new patient who came in for a LipiFlow procedure (see Common Treatments chapter) from two hours away but she had a large neurotrophic ulcer which she could not feel. She just felt dry. I actually ended up debriding her ulcer, placing a Prokera (see definition in Common Treatments chapter under amniotic membrane), and starting her on serum drops. She definitely could not feel her melting cornea, but she knew her eyes were "dry." With proper treatment, we were able to save her affected eye. She did not need a LipiFlow treatment at all. She is still on serum drops years later, and I watch her closely (every three months or so). I've had other neurotrophic keratitis patients come in with melting corneal ulcers who just felt "dry" and just cannot feel the level of damage they have in their eyes.

Neurotrophic keratitis (NK) can also have many causes, including diabetes, damage to the nerves in the eyelids after eyelid lift surgeries (blepharoplasty), autoimmune diseases like lupus, rheumatoid arthritis, as well as some infectious causes like herpetic eye disease (both from shingles or the herpes virus). Another term that has been used to describe patients with dry eye is discordant dry eye, where the cornea and eye exam look normal, but the patient has significant symptoms of dry eye disease. It is on the other end of the spectrum from traditional neurotrophic keratitis, where patients lose sensation but develop significant dry eye signs and even corneal melts.

Another more superficial version of painful dry eye is called recurrent erosion syndrome. There are a few predisposing factors, including severe dry eye, a corneal condition called anterior basement membrane dystrophy (ABMD), or a prior superficial trauma like from a fingernail or paper, all of which can lead to erosions of your corneal epithelium (the most superficial layer of your cornea). Once the corneal epithelium is injured, sometimes the attachments of the superficial layer to the basement membrane layer are not as strong as they were before. Then, when you are sleeping, and your basal tear secretion rate decreases, your eyelid sticks to your eye. Then, when you open your eyes, usually you have sharp pain, sometimes feeling like something is in your eye or rocks are in your eye. The eyelid sticking to the eyeball literally causes a mini abrasion/erosion when you open your eyes. It can be a micro-erosion which heals in 30 minutes with some watering or a significant erosion showing up like a corneal abrasion when you go to your eye doctor, which will need some lubricating or antibiotic ointment to help it heal over 1–3 days. We will talk about some patient cases later in the book where a patient was treated for regular dry eye when they really needed a different treatment for recurrent erosions to feel better.

There are also serious causes of eye pain, like glaucoma, which can cause serious irreversible damage to your optic nerve. There are two main types of glaucoma: open-angle glaucoma and narrow-angle glaucoma. The type you have depends on the configuration of the front of your eye in the angle and your eye pressure as well as optic nerve damage. With a narrow angle configuration, the angle can close intermittently, which blocks the drainage system (or trabecular meshwork) inside your eye and results in eye pain, blurry vision, halos around lights, headaches, nausea/vomiting and/or brow pain. I don't want to ignore checking for this, even if it may be obvious that dry eye disease is the cause of your symptoms. Another common cause of eye pain is referred eye pain from sinus disease. During allergy season, especially here in Virginia where I'm located, almost half of the patients who come in for eye pain have a sinus infection or dry sinuses which cause referred eye pain.

"DOC, MY CONTACTS ARE STUCK TO MY EYE."

Dry eye patients can also develop contact lens intolerance, where they cannot wear their contact lenses (CL) anymore due to irritation, redness, a history of corneal ulcers, or simply feeling like their contact lenses are stuck to their eyes when it is time to take them out. CL overwear can also cause giant papillary conjunctivitis, where the conjunctiva under the lids develops a cobblestone (bumpy) appearance and produces more inflammatory chemicals, which can worsen dry eyes. Continuing to ignore signs of CL intolerance can also lead to severe corneal infections or ulcers, which can lead to vision loss. Rarely do the surface changes progress so much that I have to tell patients that they can never wear contact lenses again. Many of the treatments we will discuss also help with CL intolerance.

"DOC, MY EYES ARE ITCHY, NOT DRY."

Eyes with dryness and inflammation can also feel "sticky." Allergies and allergic inflammation can also cause this sticky feeling which causes tear film dysfunction and leads to dry eye disease. Allergies can also cause itchy eyes. Sometimes, your eyes may have allergies, and you cannot feel it in addition to the dry eye symptoms, but we can see the allergic inflammation in your conjunctiva, and treatment with an anti-allergy eye drop, which will help your dry eye disease even if your eyes are not itchy. The amount of allergy in the eye also varies by location in the country. The eyes of patients who move to Virginia, where I'm located, can suddenly become drier. "Welcome to Virginia" is a common line I use to describe the significant effect of regional allergies on their eyes, and sinuses, and as a cause of their new dry eye disease. Traveling to other parts of the country or world on vacation can show you that it is, in fact, environmental for a lot of patients. I've never had anyone move away from Virginia due to dry eye disease, but it could be a consideration for some patients if it is a huge factor for their eyes.

"DOC, I HAVE A STYE." (YES, IT'S A SIGN OF DRY EYE.)

If you have ever had a stye or a chalazion, it could be a precursor sign of dry eye disease. If you work on the computer often, you can have a variant of dry eye disease called computer fatigue syndrome. We'll talk more about the meibomian glands in the exam section. However, you have glands in your eyelids which produce oil; these are meibomian glands (MG). If those glands get clogged and infected, we call it a stye. If the infection spreads to the whole eyelid, it is called preseptal cellulitis which looks like a swollen eyelid and you may not see the stye (inciting clogged and infected gland) until the skin infection resolves. You will need oral antibiotics if the infection gets to the cellulitis stage. Once the infection heals, but the clogged oil is still stuck in the meibomian gland, the body starts to wall it off, and you can have a chronic non-tender bump on your eyelid. We call this a chalazion (pronounced starting the same way as you say cholesterol). A chalazion can sometimes take months to go away and may need to be drained in the office. They can also cause blurry vision by pushing irregularly on your eye (and causing irregular astigmatism).

If the glands are not producing proper oil or if they are not able to squeeze out the oil at a regular rate with an average blink, then your MG can get clogged, and the surface of the eye is missing its oil layer, and this leads to dryness. The normal blink rate is reduced with any concentrated activity like computer use or reading. You can also develop small rocks in your meibomian glands called concretions. Just like you can get gallstones or kidney stones, you can get eyelid stones. You can also get stones in your lacrimal gland and lacrimal sac. Concretions can also cause pain in your eyes and corneal abrasions. I've even seen them cause a large scratch on the eye or a corneal abrasion. Removing concretions can help your eyes feel more normal and make a huge difference in your overall eye comfort, so it's important to see a dry eye specialist like me. MG research is changing how to treat dry eyes.

"DOC, THERE'S SOMETHING IN MY EYE."

Many aspects of dry eye disease can make it feel like there is something in your eyes. We've already talked about concretions and styes. If the ocular surface is damaged or the tear film is missing, the corneal cells will send a pain signal and make it feel like something is in your eyes. Over time, a callous can form on the corneal surface, which we call a Salzmann's nodule. This can also occur after a trauma to the eye as well. I have one patient with focal conjunctivochalasis (CCH) (extra loose skin on the surface of the eye, see more in the exam section) and adjacent to this area, she has a large Salzmann's nodule. I believe the CCH lead to her Salzmann's nodule. If you read about Salzmann's nodules, the cause is unclear, but I have seen it develop and cause even more irregularity of the ocular surface—as now there's a little mountain on the cornea which doesn't allow the distribution of the tears to be normal, and therefore can exacerbate dry eye disease. I have also seen it decrease with different treatments.

"DOC, MY EYE WATERS. HOW IS IT DRY?"

One confusing symptom of dry eye is watery eyes. In this situation, the surface of the eyes is not getting the nutrients it needs, so it makes extra watery tears, but those tears are not the right *quality* to help the ocular surface. Your eyes need the right quality and quantity of tears to not have dry eye disease. Emotional or crying tears also don't have the same nutritional content as normal tears. I often hear people tell me that they cry all the time, "How are my eyes dry?" But once you understand that emotional tears are not the same as your normal baseline tears, it makes more sense. I also have patients who are so dry that they cannot cry.

There is an important question to answer when your eyes are watery. Are they watering because they are making too much water (from irritation/allergies), or are they not draining enough water (the tear ducts are blocked or not in the right position against the eye like an ectropion)? Figuring out the cause of your watering eyes as a blocked tear duct is a whole different treatment than an irritation. Most patients will have irritation when in any windy situation. It is normal. If the watering is only from one eye, then it makes me strongly suspect a tear duct issue, and I'll flush the tear ducts with a small cannula in the office. Sometimes, that's enough to cure the watering if that is the cause. Treating with nasal sprays can also help. Sometimes, I need to send patients to the oculoplastic doctor for tear duct surgery to open up the tear ducts to get rid of the watering. Sometimes, when we treat dry eyes, the watering improves. It just depends on the cause of your watery eyes.

"DOC, MY EYES ARE LIGHT-SENSITIVE."

I often have patients who are so light-sensitive from dry eye disease that they can't walk outside or sit in my exam room without sunglasses. In fact, I was one of those people when my dry eye was not adequately treated in my 20s. I couldn't stand a sunny day or imagine going to the beach for enjoyment with all the sun and wind making my eyes miserable. Perhaps the corneal nerve damage over time leads to severe light sensitivity and even pain from bright lights. Dry eye with a lack of nutrition to the corneal epithelial cells leads to corneal nerve damage over time. Some treatments can help this, which we will cover in the treatments section, so don't lose hope. I can now tolerate the sun much better than I did when I was in my 20s.

This leads to the classic question of which came first. Did the dry eye cause the pain and headache (which was true for me)? Or did the migraine and headache cause abnormal nerves which led to dry eye disease? There was a review showing a much higher odds ratio of dry eye disease in migraine patients (OR=1.42–1.97 depending on whether an inpatient or outpatient setting) (Chen et al.).

Many other serious medical conditions cause light sensitivity, like uveitis or iritis, so please see your local eye doctor and do not assume it is dry eye disease. The uvea is the colored part of your eye, including the iris, ciliary body, and choroid. Uveitis is an inflammation of those parts of the eye and can cause light sensitivity. Many autoimmune diseases and infectious diseases cause uveitis including rheumatoid arthritis, ankylosing spondylitis (HLA-B27 positive), lupus, herpes, lyme disease, sarcoidosis, tuberculosis, syphilis, and many others. I recently saw a patient with bilateral panu-veitis (inflammation in the front and back of their eyes) from a recent COVID-19 infection. That is why we are here—to help you! Please do not self-treat your symptoms only and go see your local eye doctor especially if you have light sensitivity.

2

MEDICAL HISTORY QUESTIONS

PLAYING DETECTIVE AS A DOCTOR

When patients come to see me for any of the common symptoms of dry eye disease, I'm ready to play detective and figure out the cause. After listening to what's bothering patients, my first question is almost always, **"When were you last normal?"** This is not to be funny but to truly find out how long their eyes have been dry. The patient who had pink eye two months ago and now has horrible dry eyes is a whole different workup and treatment plan than someone who has had dry eyes for years.

WHEN ARE YOUR SYMPTOMS THE WORST? WHAT ENVIRONMENTAL FACTORS ARE CONTRIBUTING?

I want to know **when** your eyes are dry too.

- Are they dry all day long?
- Are they worse at the end of the day after working all day on the computer?
- Are they worse on weekdays compared to weekends when you are not in front of the computer?
- What is your blink rate?
- Are they worse when walking outside in the wind, and then they are watery?
- Are they worse right after waking up?
- Do you have sharp pain in your eyes when waking up?
- Do you sleep with your eyes open, or do you sleep with something like a CPAP or BiPAP machine blowing air on your eyes all night long?
- Do you have thyroid disease and cannot close your eyes all the way?
- Are they more irritated after a long day of wearing your contact lenses?
- Are they worse after a particular type of rice-based foundation powder that you picked up, especially to use for a luncheon with your friends (yes, this happened to a patient who was well controlled until one Sunday afternoon)?

- Do you use an eyelash growth serum? Note: Certain lash growth serums also have a medication (prostaglandin analog) that can cause your meibomian glands to be dysfunctional, contributing to dry eye disease and causing some orbital fat atrophy over time which can make your eyes look sunken in over time.
- Have you been on isotretinoin (used for severe acne) in the past?
- Do you have mucus coming out of your eyes, and do you use a tissue or Q-tip to pull the mucus out? This can cause *"mucus fishing syndrome"* with even more mucus and eye irritation. Please don't do this. Please talk to your eye doctor about what you may be putting on your eyes and how you're taking care of them to make sure you are not exacerbating the situation.

You may have seen the **SPEED questionnaire** asking about your symptoms. The SPEED questionnaire asks you about "Dryness, Grittiness or Scratchiness, Soreness or Irritation, Burning or Watering Eye Fatigue" and the frequency and severity of each symptom. There's also the **Ocular Surface Disease Index (OSDI) questionnaire** which asks about the frequency of your symptoms, including your light sensitivity, eyes feeling gritty, painful, blurry vision, poor vision, trouble with activities of daily living (ADLs) like reading, driving, working on the computer or watching TV and if they worsen with wind, low humidity or air-conditioned areas. Both the SPEED and OSDI questionnaires are used in clinical practice and medical studies to demonstrate improvement in dry eye with different treatments or interventions. It can be useful for monitoring your dry eyes with a score as well. I generally ask my patients with each visit what percent improvement they have with whatever treatment we did to help me gauge what I need to do next.

WHAT MEDICAL CONDITIONS DO YOU HAVE WHICH CAN AFFECT YOUR EYES?

Do you have medical conditions which can make you more prone to dry eyes, like thyroid eye disease with prominent eyes (what we call proptosis or exophthalmos)? Do you have neurological diseases which prevent you from blinking normally, like Parkinson's disease or a rare mitochondrial myopathy that can cause CPEO (chronic progressive external ophthalmoplegia)? Did you have a stroke or have Bell's palsy, causing facial paralysis and the inability to close your eyes fully? Do you have a strict or limited diet that has led to vitamin A deficiency and caused decreased night vision as well as dry eye disease? Believe it or not, it is not just a third-world disease. I have diagnosed this at least twice in the last ten years here in Virginia. The three major diseases that contribute to dry eye disease are autoimmune diseases like rheumatoid arthritis or lupus, thyroid disease, and sleep apnea in my patients. One autoimmune disease to highlight is Sjogren's disease when the patient usually has dry eyes and dry mouth. Hormonal changes also play a factor. We'll talk more about this in the Lifestyle Medicine section.

HISTORY OF REFRACTIVE SURGERY OR OTHER EYE SURGERY

Many types of refractive surgery, some more than others, can cause worsening dry eye disease. The main ones known to most people are LASIK or PRK. There is also refractive lens exchange surgery or ICL. In LASIK (laser-assisted in situ keratomileusis), a flap is created in the cornea, and a laser is used to basically laser your glasses prescription onto your cornea. PRK (photorefractive keratectomy) is just like LASIK except there is no corneal flap. Thus, PRK is thought to be safer if you may be exposed to trauma, and it is safer in dry eye predisposed patients as the corneal nerves are not cut, whereas in LASIK they are cut with the flap creation. A prior surgery called RK (radial keratectomy) also contributed to some dry eye and does commonly result in fluctuating vision during the day. Intraocular surgery, like cataract surgery or refractive lens exchange surgery, or ICL (implantable collamer lenses) placed in the eye, can be a contributing factor to dry eye, especially in someone predisposed to dry eye for other reasons. Surgeries where the conjunctiva (where mucin-producing goblet cells live) is disrupted, like retinal surgeries with scleral buckles or eye muscle surgeries, sometimes predispose patients to dry eye disease. These are all successful surgeries, and most patients do not have problems after these surgeries. However, some people are predisposed to dry eye disease due to other factors, and these surgeries can exacerbate their condition significantly.

HOW OFTEN ARE YOU USING ARTIFICIAL TEARS?

I want to know if you are overusing artificial tears. I explain that just like washing your hands too much and causing "dishpan hands." If you overuse artificial tears, you can wash away your healthy nutrients and oils on the ocular surface and cause yourself to have dry or *dishpan eyes.*" I recommend only using regular artificial tears a maximum of four times per day if needed. Regular artificial tears also have a preservative that can cause dry eye disease. <u>Overusing tears is the one thing that can make you worse than you realize</u>. If you have dry eye disease, I will likely switch you to a preservative-free artificial tear drop but still limit your use of these to no more than four times per day. If you feel like you need them more, we need to do additional therapies to get you better.

Sometimes, the patient doesn't know exactly what they are doing to make it worse, so then I ask them to keep a journal.

A medical journal of symptoms and days and times when they are worse helps them, and helps me, as the doctor, know the cause and figure out a better treatment plan. This is true for many medical conditions, not just dry eyes.

3

THE DRY EYE EXAM

YOUR OVERALL APPEARANCE

When you see your eye doctor, they are not just doing tests. They are looking at everything. Part of the regular medical exam is looking at the patient's external appearance as well as their gait when walking into the room to see if there are any neurological signs, such as a shuffling gait, like Parkinson's, or paralysis of your face or body.

THE EXTERNAL EXAM

When we look at your face for the "external exam," we are looking for facial asymmetry as well. It was somewhat more challenging with the mask we wore during the COVID-19 pandemic, but sometimes, I would ask patients to take their masks off to look at their whole facial appearance. Sometimes I ask them to stick their tongue out and do other parts of the neurological exam, like checking their hearing or facial muscles for strength and symmetry to check for stroke. With the external exam, I'm also looking for exophthalmos, the medical word for prominent eyeballs. There is a way we can even measure this (with a Hertel exophthalmometer). I ask patients to close their eyes and look and see if their eyelids are fully closed. Sometimes there are apparent signs of meibomian gland dysfunction, like styes (infected red bumps) or chalazion (hard, non-tender bumps) on the eyelids.

WE CANNOT IGNORE THE AREA AROUND OUR EYES

Another part of the exam is tapping on the sinuses and nasolacrimal duct area to evaluate for sinus disease or any lacrimal sac infection. There are many places where I evaluate eye pain by tapping on the forehead for the frontal sinus, the cheeks for the maxillary sinus, and the inner corners of the eyes for the ethmoid sinuses. I also check the area of the supraorbital and infraorbital notches on the orbital rim (the bony part around your eye) to check for any hypersensitivity to the nerves and any pain there, which could be triggering eye pain but not be related to dry eye disease. Patients with nerve tenderness around the orbit also can have tenderness on the back of their head. This location

on the back of the skull is where the greater and lesser occipital nerves come out of the skull. These nerves can become
inflamed or compressed and trigger pain. This is called
occipital neuralgia. I also look for a rash like the one seen in
shingles or an allergic reaction on your face. Eyelid swelling
can also be linked to other skin infections and allergies.

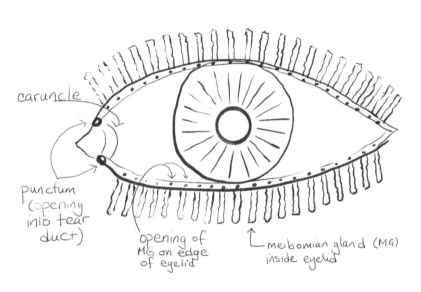

Diagram #1

THE SLIT LAMP OR BIOMICROSCOPE EXAM

Once I am examining patients with the slit lamp microscope
for the eye exam, I look systematically at the eye to not miss
anything. We are taught to look at the lashes, the meibomian
glands, the puncta (opening of the tear ducts), the lacrimal
gland, the tear film, the conjunctiva (both on the inside of the
eyelid as well as on the eyeball above the sclera or the white

part of the eye), the cornea, and a quick look inside the eye for any inflammation, check your angles or other causes of blurry vision like cataracts, glaucoma or macular degeneration. However, we're not going to go through the entire list of problems that goes through my head when I'm looking at a patient's main complaint.

EYELASHES ARE SO IMPORTANT!

When I'm looking at the eyelashes, I'm looking for any blepharitis (crusting of the eyelashes), evidence of Demodex (a little mite that lives in a patient's eyelashes and skin), or folliculitis (a skin infection around an eyelash follicle). Regular blepharitis (from skin bacteria), as well as seborrheic blepharitis (sometimes linked to a skin fungal infection), is also important to diagnose correctly and treat.

When I'm looking at the meibomian glands (the things that look like fat eyelashes per my daughter in my diagram #1), I examine the opening of the gland and see if they are capped and look at the MG anatomy on a scanning test like the LipiScan (structure of the gland), and I push gently to see what kind of oil is expressed from the gland (function of the gland). A clogged gland can also cause a foreign body sensation. There have been many patients who come in with focal pain, and I press on the eyelid releasing a clogged gland, and they feel much better. You can do a manual expression of the eyelid glands after warm compresses if you feel comfortable, but I do not advise this routinely as I prefer your glands work on their own, and I worry about you poking your eye accidentally.

I can also see fine blood vessels on the lid margin that shouldn't be there (telangiectasias), and their presence can signal the start of "ocular rosacea" and inflammation of the meibomian glands (Tavassoli et al.). I've also seen them sometimes develop in patients on certain glaucoma eye drops (the prostaglandin analogs (PGAs) like latanoprost, travoprost, bimatoprost, and tafluprost), and it has been shown that these eyedrops can cause meibomian gland dysfunction.

DEMODEX BLEPHARITIS

A diagnosis of Demodex is always shocking to my patients. We have many organisms living on us and inside of us. Some are beneficial to us, like your good gut bacteria. Some are not, like Demodex. Yes, I can see the little mite tails and eggs on your eyelashes. If you want to see them, I usually remove an eyelash and put it on a slide, and show you under the regular microscope right there in my clinic. Just because you have Demodex blepharitis does not mean you have to treat it. Some sources say we all have Demodex on our skin. Demodex can also live in your makeup (we will talk more about this later).

However, if Demodex mites are contributing to your dry eye disease, styes, chalazion, or folliculitis, it is essential to get this appropriately treated. I've had patients with chronic skin ulcerations on their legs or scalp who I have diagnosed with Demodex, switched them to a tea tree cleanser, and have them switch their shampoo or soap to one with tea tree oil too. They come back and tell me their leg or scalp lesion is gone too, when prior treatments by their other doctors have not helped, and the tea tree oil soap/shampoo can be curative. Tea tree oil has been shown to be effective in controlling but not eradicating Demodex mites (Koo et al., Savla et al.), but do not put the full concentration near your eye, only the 1–2% as found in the tea tree eyelid cleanser (see treatment section). A tiny little mite can have such a huge impact. I have also had patients reinfect themselves if they allow a pet or untreated partner to share their pillow. We'll talk more about the treatment later.

LOOKING AT YOUR TEAR DUCT SYSTEM

When I look at the punctum or the opening of the tear duct in the middle corner of the eye, I'm looking for the size of the tear duct opening, especially if you have watery eyes. If your punctum is small or has purulent discharge with a chronic infection or rocks in your tear ducts/sac, this could be the cause of your watery eyes. If indicated, I will flush your tear ducts to test for obstruction or stenosis of your nasolacrimal duct, which may contribute to watery eyes. If there is an obstruction, sometimes flushing the tear duct system can be diagnostic and also therapeutic, as we talked about briefly in the "watery eye" symptom section. I have seen one patient who had rheumatoid arthritis, had chronic dacryocystitis (tear duct infection), and even perforated her cornea from a combination of her rheumatoid inflammation, tear duct debris, inflammation, and severe dry eye disease. The position of the lower eyelid and the puncta is important. If your eyelids are loose or turned out (ectropion), then the puncta is not touching the eye like it should be, and the tears cannot get into the tear ducts, so they overflow causing watery eyes. We can test the lower eyelid with the snapback test.

Some strange cases I've seen include a patient with eye pain but who had an eyelash embedded in his tear duct chronically scratching his eye (until I removed it) as well as patients with eyelashes embedded within scar tissues inside the eyelid as well in folds of the conjunctiva (common if you have had eye surgery where the conjunctiva was cut). Sometimes we just have to look for strange causes of eye pain in strange locations of the eye.

THE LACRIMAL GLAND VERSUS THE LACRIMAL SAC

I will look at the lacrimal gland more closely if you have a complaint of pain in that area or a droopy upper outer eyelid. I have seen many cases of lacrimal gland involvement of another process, like cancer of the lacrimal gland or sarcoidosis, but, generally, its appearance does not change in dry eye disease. The lacrimal gland contributes to normal tear production but goes into hyper-mode in emotional tears, like when you are crying. It is easy to get the lacrimal gland, lacrimal sac, and nasolacrimal duct confused in location and their effect on dry eye disease. Please look at diagram #2 below to see the different locations.

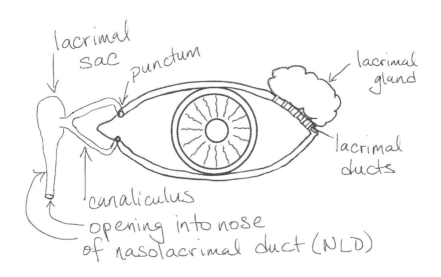

Diagram #2

THE TEAR FILM

I look at the tear film on the eyelid margin before moving the eyelid. The tear film should be clear and abundant (about 1 mm in height). If there are foamy tears with little soap bubbles (saponification), we know there is some meibomian gland dysfunction and abnormal oil on the ocular surface.

We will come back to look at the tear film differently in a few paragraphs during the exam section.

THE MEIBOMIAN GLANDS AND ROCKS IN YOUR EYELIDS (CONCRETIONS)

When I look at the conjunctiva on the inside of the eyelid, I am looking at the meibomian glands again to see if there are any structural changes or concretions which can form in the meibomian gland. Sometimes an area where the meibomian glands have died looks darker or pinker than the rest of the inside of the eyelid. Some patients can feel the concretions significantly, and some cannot. I do remove concretions if the patient has sandy or gritty feelings in their eyes. Otherwise, I tend to leave them alone. Sometimes, patients have used Q-tips to sweep under their own eyelids at home or inside their lower lid trying to remove a foreign body, but this can aggravate the concretion and cause the overlying conjunctiva to become abraded, and then they can feel the concretion even more (until I remove it). Please do not try to sweep under your eyelids. Use eye wash (available in your local stores) to irrigate your eye if needed.

We can also image the meibomian glands with many different devices, including the LipiScan or LipiView, which uses infrared meibography. I like to use it for patient education as well as determining what therapy you may need. One unexpected fact is that high blood sugar, like in diabetes, can cause dysfunction of your meibomian glands, too (see Lifestyle Medicine section on sugar).

THE CONJUNCTIVA

Then I look at the conjunctiva on the eyeball, looking for any other causes of irritation like calcium deposits within the conjunctiva, pinguecula, pterygium (which grow onto the cornea as well), or any signs of OSSN (ocular surface squamous neoplasia—cancer on the surface of the eye which I definitely do not want to miss). I look at the cornea for any punctate keratitis (dry spots on the cornea). Just like you can see dry skin on your arms or legs, or feet, I can see dry spots from dryness and damage on the corneal surface. As mentioned prior, I look inside the eye for any anterior chamber inflammation, checking for the anterior chamber depth (for narrow angles) and intraocular lens clarity. The anterior chamber is the space between the cornea and the iris.

There's another condition called SLK (superior limbic keratoconjunctivitis), where the superior part of the conjunctiva under the eyelids becomes loose and overrides on itself, and becomes chronically irritated. It can be associated with thyroid disease, rheumatoid arthritis, dry eye, floppy eyelid syndrome, allergic conjunctivitis, trachoma, prior viral conjunctivitis, and contact lens overwear. So it is important to look at the conjunctiva under the eyelid on the eyeball and also to evert the eyelids to look at the conjunctiva on the back side of the upper eyelid.

Conjunctivochalasis (CCH) is a condition where you can get redundant conjunctiva which can override itself as well as the cornea with each blink and cause eye pain and a foreign body sensation. It is sometimes called "mechanical dry eye." Sometimes patients with CCH feel better in a contact lens on their eye because the contact lens pushes the extra conjunctiva away from the cornea, and the patient doesn't feel the subsequent irritation anymore. The CCH could also impact the goblet cell basal tear production. The chronic rubbing from the extra conjunctiva on itself could create inflammation as well. I have also seen CCH in an area of Salzmann's nodular degeneration of the cornea (kind of like a callous) superonasal which is interesting as it makes you wonder if the cause of the Salzmann's nodular degeneration is from the CCH and chronic rubbing/irritation. It is believed to be age-related, but rubbing your eyes could contribute as well, so please don't rub your eyes. Typically CCH is seen inferiorly but SLK could be a variant of CCH but superiorly. The underlying causes are not well understood.

FLOPPY EYELID SYNDROME AND LOOSE EYELIDS

This is another interesting condition basically caused by eyelid rubbing either by the patient or the pillow inadvertently when sleeping with your face/eyes against the pillow.

The tissues can become so loose that they can evert (flip inside out) with mild pressure and do so when you're asleep and can become irritated with exposure all night. Floppy eyelid syndrome can also be exacerbated by sleep apnea as well as by sleeping with a CPAP machine. The mechanism is thought to be the chronic air forcing the eyelids open at night as well as other unknown factors. If the eyelids are extremely loose, sometimes they require surgery to tighten. If the lower eyelid is not in the proper position, too loose and not opposed to the eye (ectropion), or too loose, and the eyelid is turning in (entropion), both can cause irritation of the eye and watering and dry eye symptoms.

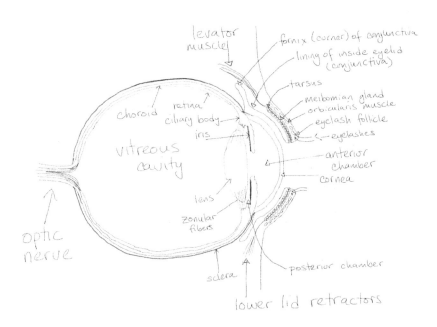

Diagram #3

THE CORNEA AND CORNEAL DYES
(FLUORESCEIN, ETC.)

The "eyes are the windows to the soul" (Shakespeare), and the light has to go through the cornea to reach the retina for you to see properly. The cornea is the clear window over the iris, which is where you place a contact lens if you wear contact lenses. It is an amazing part of the body as it is one of the only parts of our bodies which is CLEAR! When the cornea is damaged from dry eye disease, it can become scarred and cloudy. It can also have ulcers and nerve damage. Sometimes we can even see the corneal nerves with the biomicroscope and definitely with confocal microscopy imaging. The limbus (the area where the sclera meets the cornea) holds the limbal stem cells. These cells are responsible for healing damaged corneas. However, if the feedback loop is damaged, or the limbal stem cells are damaged, they cannot heal the damaged cornea, and this can lead to a downward spiral feedback loop which can worsen dry eye disease. It is important to check corneal sensation (can you actually feel damage to your cornea?), especially if the amount of damage I see is out of proportion to the pain you are feeling (either too much or too little). There are a few different ways to check corneal sensation, but the most common would be with a wisp of cotton from a sterile Q-tip in the clinic. Corneal damage with limbal stem cell damage can show a whorl or swirl pattern of damage on the cornea as well.

Chronic blepharitis (or crusting of the eyelashes) can also cause damage to the cornea ranging from mild infections/inflammations like staphylococcal marginal keratitis (corneal infection near the limbus) to full-on blepharoconjunctivitis with scar tissue and blood vessel overgrowth over the entire cornea which can impact your vision. Simply cleaning your eyelashes can have a huge impact on your cornea, your vision, and your dry eye disease (read more in the treatment section).

Next, I usually instill a numbing drop with some fluorescein dye (the stuff that turns your tears orange for a few minutes) into the eye and look at your tear film and the corneal surface. It can highlight subtle irregularities in the corneal surface, such as subclinical ABMD (anterior basement membrane dystrophy), which can cause irregular tear distribution and cause more blurry vision than we would expect. I also look and count the tear break-up time (TBUT), or how fast the tear film breaks up over the surface of the eye, and this may be the most predictive test to tell us if you have dry eye disease (Rege et al.). Normal TBUT is over 15 seconds, and that helps me know how healthy the tear film concentration is. I also look at how much dye sits on the eye/eyelid margin. Is it too much and not draining down the tear duct fast enough? The fluorescein dye also stains or highlights damaged areas of the cornea or areas missing normal epithelial cells. Another dye we can use is rose bengal, which helps stain dead cells, especially if they are not protected by the mucin in the tear film. Yet another dye is lissamine green, which can complement the fluorescein dye test by staining abnormal epithelial (surface) cells on both the cornea and conjunctiva (whereas fluorescein stains areas without cells). The most common way of evaluating damage is still fluorescein dye in your doctor's office.

THE SCHIRMER'S TEST – STRIPS OF PAPER IN YOUR EYELID

For most dry eye patients, we use the Schirmer's test to evaluate how many tears you make in five minutes using the capillary action properties of water on paper. I usually use the version where I numb your eyes with a numbing eyedrop, wait about one minute, put the strips of paper (specific tear flow test strips) in your lower lids, and start my timer. During the 5-minute test, I'm usually telling patients all about dry eye treatment options and giving them information. I wait one minute before starting to make sure we don't have a false result from the numbing drop volume itself. Another option is drying the inside of the eyelid with a cotton-tipped applicator (CTA or Q-tip) before starting the test.

There are actually a few different ways of doing a Schirmer's test. Technically, the test I'm doing in the clinic is the basal tear secretion or production test, as the numbing drops should negate any reflex tearing you may have from the strips of paper in your eyelid. You can have the test done without any numbing medication (Schirmer's type I) or without any numbing and tickling inside your nose with a CTA (nasal stimulation with Schirmer's type II). The official Schirmer's type I and II include both reflex tearing and basal tear production (your normal rate of tear production). Normal results are 15 mm or more on the paper strip for the basal tear secretion test. Less than 10 mm is abnormal, and less than 5 mm indicates significant dry eye, which needs to be treated. Treatments like prescription drops get approved by the FDA by demonstrating an improvement in the Schirmer's scores over weeks to months. Some patients even have a Schirmer's score of zero, so they make zero tears over the 5-minute testing window.

TEAR OSMOLARITY TEST

Osmolarity tells us the chemical composition of your tears as a number. We have a way to test tear osmolarity with a machine from TearLab, now called Trukera. They have a handheld device that can sample some of your tears in the office, and the machine can tell us your osmolarity. I simplify it by saying it tells me how salty or concentrated your tears are compared to normal. I do find the test somewhat useful, but it doesn't change my management, so I stopped using the tests and machine recently. Your eye doctor may find the information helps steer their treatment more, and it can also serve as a mode of measuring your success with the treatment chosen.

4

COMMON AND UNCOMMON TREATMENTS

STARTING WITH THE ABCS

When I say start with the ABCs for the treatment of dry eye disease, I'm talking about:

A – Avoiding things that dry you out
B – Basic over-the-counter treatments
C – Consult your local eye doctor if that's not enough

For my patients, *my goal is to normalize and optimize the ocular surface, so they don't think about their eyes all the time. Their eyes become a regular part of their body again.* When patients return for follow-up, I ask them to quantify their improvement as a percentage which helps guide me as to how much more I need to do to help them. You can write down your improvements as a percentage in your medical journal to help you track how much better or worse you are with each therapy. I approach the treatment of dry eye with a minimalist approach and try to use the bare minimum therapy needed to get you feeling normal again. For some of you, it may be a simple change, and for others, you may need many therapies for some time to get you back to normal.

ENVIRONMENTAL CHANGES, SCREEN TIME, AND SCREEN MODIFICATIONS

When we talked about the detective list of questions, changing some of your environment can have a considerable impact on your dry eye disease. The basic rules I tell all patients are (1) to avoid having the vent pointing toward their face or eyes when in the car, especially during the winter with the dry heat; (2) to have an anti-glare screen on their computer monitor; (3) to set their computer screen and phone to night shift mode (blue-blocking and slightly yellow/orange) and dark mode (black background to help contrast sensitivity and vision)); and (4) to monitor their work and sleep environment to have a humidifier if needed and not to have a fan blowing on their face.

Another good rule to follow is the 20–20–20 rule: take a break every 20 minutes and look away 20 feet for 20 seconds. This helps eye fatigue with computer use or near work as well as prevents the progression of myopia (nearsightedness) by helping break your accommodation of your ciliary body muscles.

If you're waking up with painful dry eyes, other options are: 1) wear a mask when sleeping; 2) use a lubricating ointment before sleeping; and 3) buy a specialized eye mask that can fully seal around your eyes if you are sleeping with a CPAP or BiPAP machine such as the EyeSeals 4.0 from Eye Eco. It helps block out the air from the machine, which may be blowing on your eyes all night.

DAILY MODIFICATIONS

Contact Lenses

In dry eye, one simple modification that can help is changing the monthly or two-weekly contact lens to a daily contact lens. The daily lenses are much thinner and allow the tear film to penetrate the contact and nourish the cornea more. The anterior ⅓ of the cornea only gets its nutrition from the tears. The posterior ⅔ of the cornea gets its nutrition from the fluid inside of the eye. You will also hopefully eliminate sleeping in your contact lenses. Sleeping in your contact lenses is the number one cause of a corneal ulcer. Please don't do this. Other treatment options we will talk about also help contact lens intolerance, including serum drops, IPL, and treating allergic changes in your eyes.

Makeup

Another simple modification is changing your makeup (you can figure out which one is making you worse by keeping a medical journal) and taking off your makeup at night every single night. Sometimes, I see patients with beige makeup (usually powder) floating in their tear film and actually embedded under their conjunctiva under their eyelids. Most of these patients do have dry eye disease, but I don't check all normal patients by flipping or everting their eyelids to check underneath, so I cannot be sure. There is no way for me to remove this embedded makeup. I want to educate you to close your eyes before applying the powder makeup to your face. I haven't seen eyeliner or mascara embedded in the eyelid conjunctiva as much.

Most people do remove makeup daily, but some don't, and I want to remind you it is for the benefit of your eyes to do this. Please use a specific eye makeup remover. Many beauty makeup companies have eye makeup removers. Some of my favorites are Mary Kay's makeup remover and Arbonne's eye makeup remover. Some patients who are sensitive to eye makeup removers can use coconut oil or argan oil to soften the makeup and then completely remove it. Many companies sell over-the-counter eyelid wipes, which are able to remove makeup as well, like OCuSOFT or OCuSOFT Plus. Eye Eco's Tea Tree cleanser also removes makeup and can help kill Demodex in the process. (See the eyelid wipes section below.)

It is also important to change your makeup regularly. The general recommendation is to replace your makeup when you replace your toothbrush, every three months or so. This includes eyeliner and mascara. Demodex mites/eggs can live in the makeup as well, and you can re-infect yourself. If you are actively treating yourself for Demodex blepharitis, you can use disposable wands to clean the base of the lashes to get the crusting off (a tip taught to me by a patient). You can also use these disposable wands to apply a few wands of mascara for an important event. Remember, no double dipping, or you will contaminate your new mascara again with the Demodex mite.

Quality Sleep

Another critical factor that contributes to dry eye is the amount of sleep you get overnight. We know from sleep science that excess screen time one hour before sleep can disrupt your circadian rhythm. You need to put away all electronic devices and turn the TV off at least one hour prior to sleep and develop a healthier bedtime routine. Lifestyle Medicine also tells us we need 7–9 hours of sleep every night. I have so many patients who tell me they are sleeping at 2 or 3 a.m. and falling asleep watching television. Then, they wake up with dry eyes and painful eyes. I've also had patients who may drink some alcohol (even a small amount) later at night, not get enough sleep, and wake up with a large scratch on their eyes (corneal abrasion) from sleeping with their eyes open. Not only is sleep critical to your overall health, but it is also important for your eye health.

Essential Omega-3s

Once we have looked at your environment and sleep, let's turn to omegas. There are many types of omegas on the market, including omega-3s, omega-6s, and omega-9s. Our bodies need all of them, but we don't get enough omega-3s in our diet. So, we need to supplement with either a dietary source intentionally every day or with a supplement.

Omega-3s are commonly supplemented with fish oil. There are many versions of fish oil, but our bodies better able to absorb the natural triglyceride (TG) form of omega-3s than the ethyl ester (EE) form found in most fish oils on the market. There are also three forms of omega-3s: EPA, DHA, and ALA. Fish usually convert the ALA form to the EPA and DHA form for us, and we are better able to utilize that form. The DHA form is also essential for brain health as we age to help decrease the risk of dementia and helps the baby's brain develop better in utero (I took higher doses of DHA when I was pregnant for this reason).

There are many different vegan sources of omega-3s as well, including walnuts, hemp seeds, chia seeds, olive oil, algae oil, flaxseed, brussels sprouts, and perilla oil. Most vegan sources of omega-3s are in the ALA form, and our bodies need to convert that to the DHA or EPA form for us to get the maximum benefit. You can remember that walnuts look like a "little brain" to remember that they have omega-3s which can help your brain and eyes. There's also a supplement with GLA with EPA (HydroEye) that may help some patients with dry eye disease. Different patients respond to different sources of omega-3s. Some only tolerate vegan sources, and they do help with dry eye disease.

Overall, I recommend a minimum of 800–1,000 mg of omega-3s per day in most adults (as recommended by the American Heart Association to lower blood pressure, risk of stroke, high cholesterol, and high triglycerides) and double that dose if you have moderate to severe dry eyes for at least 3–6 months until you start feeling better. I recommend the PRN (Physician Recommended Nutriceuticals) DE3 product, either in capsules or liquid (it doesn't taste fishy to me), or the Nordic Naturals brand, which has the highest quality fish-based omega-3s on the market. Both companies also have a vegan formula of omega-3s if you prefer that. The vegan versions have algae oil and olive oil, like the Nordic Naturals vegan-friendly supplements or the PRN Omega-V. Please be sure to read all your labels correctly. Sometimes companies will advertise based on the amount of fish oil (1,000 mg) in the capsule, but the amount of omega-3s may be much lower. Make sure you are smart in the way you read supplement labels. I personally take the PRN DE3 product every day.

You may be surprised to hear this, but *almost 50% of my dry eye patients only need omega-3s to help them and no other medical treatments.* Once I get them on a high dose of omega-3s, most feel at least 50% better within 1–2 months. The other 50% will need additional therapies, which we are going to talk about more here. It makes sense when you know that omega-3s are anti-inflammatory and inflammation is one of the main causes of dry eye disease. Please read more on my website. Studies have shown a 17% lower risk of dry eye disease in women if they intake omega-3s (Miljanovic et al.). That's huge, in my opinion, and I actually think it is higher than that if you are taking the proper amount and type of omega-3s.

Omega-3s also help if you have styes and chalazions. Omega-3s will help normalize the oil secretions from the meibomian gland. They are also anti-inflammatory and will help styes and chalazions resolve faster. I had a young patient once, about eight years old, who had a large chalazion for over two years by the time his mother brought him to see me. She did not want to have it drained surgically as he would have to be under anesthesia, and it didn't appear to affect his vision. She needed a medical therapy to help him. Over the course of four months, on half a teaspoon of the PRN DE omega-3 liquid formula, the chalazion became smaller and smaller and traveled down the eyelid until it disappeared. Amazing results for a one-half teaspoon of a quality omega-3 like the PRN DE formula (see resources section) when nothing else had worked for two years prior! I've had similar results with other chalazion patients who do not want drainage of their chalazion.

BASIC EYE TREATMENTS

Artificial Tears

There are so many different types of eye drops on the market. In broad categories, there are artificial tears or lubricating drops, lubricating ointments, anti-allergy drops, and eye washes to rinse your eyes in case of emergency chemical exposure or a foreign body in your eyes. Artificial tears vary in their components and viscosity agents, ranging from having only a watery component to having various oil components, like mineral oil or flaxseed oil. Studies don't point to one being better than the other. Thicker agents hold better overnight on your eye when you are sleeping, like eye gels. Some are more soothing to certain patients than others. Therefore, trial and error is needed to determine which one your eye likes if you regularly use artificial tears.

Types of viscosity agents in artificial tears: carbomer 940 (polyacrylic acid), carboxymethyl cellulose (CMC), dextran, hyaluronic acid (HA), HP-guar, hydroxypropyl methylcellulose (HPMC), polyvinyl alcohol (PVA), polyvinylpyrrolidone (PVP) and polyethylene glycol (Jones et al. DEWS II). There's even a slow-release version that looks like a grain of rice (Lacrisert™) that patients can put inside their lower lids, and it constantly releases nourishment/lubrication to the ocular surface.

I have many patients who are overusing drops when they first come to see me. I had one lady who was using tears every 15 minutes all day long, even pulling over to the side of the road to put in drops so she could see to drive. She definitely had "dishpan eyes," which were red. She had developed corneal scarring and had a component of SLK (superior limbic keratoconjunctivitis) with loose conjunctiva from eye rubbing as well. I had her stop the drops and put her on serum drops (we will talk about this soon) every hour for 1 month before her eyes finally calmed down. We were then able to taper to 4x per day after about 3–4 months, and she's doing great now, many years later. Lesson from this case: please do not overuse artificial tears and go see your eye doctor or a dry eye specialist.

Most eye drops, unless they say they are preservative-free, have preservatives. It is well known that benzalkonium chloride (BAK), a preservative in eye drops to help prevent bacterial infection of the dropper bottle, can cause dry eye and ocular surface irritation. Most tear companies make a preservative-free (PF) version of their tears that comes in little vials rather than big bottles.

There are so many options for tears and gels, but some of my favorites are:

- Refresh Mega-3
- Refresh Optive Advanced or Optive PF
- Refresh Celluvisc PF (thicker gel drop)
- Refresh Optive Gel drops
- Refresh PM

- Systane Ultra and Systane Ultra PF
- Systane Complete and Systane Complete PF
- Theratears and Theratears PF
- Oasis Tears
- Retaine MGD PF

A couple of new products that seem promising, but I don't have much experience with yet are:

- iVizia PF
- Optase MGD or Optase Intense dry eye drops

Tip on using preservative-free vials: As long as you don't contaminate the tip of the PF vial, you can sometimes recap the vials or leave them standing up in a covered container like a clean orange normal prescription bottle from the pharmacy. Preservative-free medications help decrease your ocular toxicity significantly. Some brands have a new micro-dropper that can protect drops from infection and are in big bottles but still, PF like the Systane drops. I recommend that PF vials only be used for 24 hours at the maximum.

Red-Out Drops

Make sure you do not use the "red-out" drops too much. Those have a vasoconstrictor medication in them which makes your blood vessels shrink, and that's how they get the "red-out." But your blood vessels can get "addicted" to that medication if you use it more than 3–5 days in a row, and they will be redder when you don't use them. A new drop called "Lumify" has a different vasoconstrictor compound in a low concentration that may be safer to use daily for adults. Please do not use these medications in children without speaking to your ophthalmologist.

Anti-Allergy Eye Drops

Anti-allergy eye drops can help dry eye disease as they calm down allergic inflammation. There are many over-the-counter (OTC) anti-allergy drops, and there are many prescription ones as well. The most common component is ketotifen which is an antihistamine and can be used up to 2x per day. As with any medication, you should close your eyes for 2–3 minutes after instillation to allow the medication to absorb fully onto the surface of your eye. Some brand names of ketotifen are Zaditor and Alaway. There is also a generic version of this from your local grocery or drug store, and it is even cheaper at bulk warehouse stores like Costco. Another one is olopatadine or Pataday which is also an anti-histamine. It was a prescription drug until recently and has become OTC. It has a few different concentrations 0.1%, 0.2%, and 0.7%. The 0.1% is twice-a-day dosing, and the latter two are once-a-day dosing. Stronger is not always better. Some patients have good relief and fewer side effects with the lower concentration drops. There's also naphazoline which is in the Visine Allergy OTC.

Many prescription eye drops can help as well, including cromolyn, Lastacaft (alcaftadine)—this is now over-the-counter, Bepreve (bepotastine), Elestat (epinastine), and Optivar (azelastine). There are some more uncommon ones that I've never used before, like Emadine (emedastine), Alomide (lodoxamide), Alocril (nedocromil), and Alamast (pemirolast). Many types of topical steroids can also help with dry eye and allergies but should be used with caution as chronic steroid use can have secondary side effects. However, sometimes we do need to use steroids to calm down the eyes and allow them to respond better to other therapies.

Anti-Allergy Nasal Sprays

Many anti-allergy nasal sprays on the market can help with dry eye disease, too, by combating allergic inflammation from the nose. Remember, the eyes and the nose are connected through the lacrimal system and the sinuses. That's why when you cry, you can get a stuffy or runny nose. Simple OTC nasal saline spray can help nasal congestion and, therefore, ocular inflammation. Sometimes sinus pain is due to dry sinus passages and a saline gel nasal spray can help your eye pain as well.

There are both non-steroid anti-allergy nasal sprays and steroid nasal sprays. Many of the eye drops we've talked about are also available as nasal sprays, such as olopatadine, cromolyn, and azelastine. Many people use nasal steroids to help their allergies, such as fluticasone. But please check with your doctor as chronic use of steroids has more side effects than chronic use of anti-allergy medications, which are not steroids. I'm not a huge fan of steroid nasal sprays. Chronic use of any type of steroid can cause cataracts and your eye pressure to be elevated, which can lead to glaucoma or glaucoma progression in the future. However, if you need steroids (pills, inhaled, nasal spray, or shots) to function or breathe, then they are essential, and you need to listen to your doctors who are taking care of you.

Anti-Allergy Oral Medications

As far as oral anti-allergy medications, many are helpful, but some can also contribute to dry eye disease as they are known to worsen dry eye disease, especially if they have a decongestant component or end in "-D." The antihistamine pills that are OTC, like Claritin (loratadine), Zyrtec (cetirizine), and Allegra (fexofenadine), have all been known to worsen dry eye disease. However, they can also be tremendously helpful for dry eyes. Sometimes one of these is worse than the other in certain patients and may require trial and error to find one that does not worsen your dry eye disease. It is better not to get the one that ends in "-D" as that is even more drying to your eyes and can cause exacerbations of narrow-angle glaucoma. A prescription medication called montelukast does not usually worsen dry eye disease as much and can be helpful and is my personal favorite if you have failed the OTC medications. There's another new OTC medication called Xyzal (levocetirizine), a variant of cetirizine, which is also helpful for my patients. All anti-allergy pills can cause sleepiness, so please also monitor for that.

Eyelid Wipes and Cleansers

There are many eyelid wipes on the market these days. There are ones with soap to help you clean your eyelashes (OCuSOFT), ones with eyelid conditioners (OCuSOFT Plus), ones with coconut oil (Blephadex), some with components from okra (Zocular eyelid wipes or Zocular foaming spray— one of my patients loves this!), some with tea tree oil (Cliradex or Demodex Oust or Blephadex or from Oasis) which helps treat Demodex (Savla et al.). There are many others. My favorite is the tea tree foaming cleanser from Eye Eco, which is a 1% tea tree oil concentration and helps remove makeup and clean your lashes and kill Demodex. I really like the OCuSOFT Allergy Eyelid wipes too. It's great for my kids who hate eye drops but have significant eye allergies in the springtime.

Important Tip: It is important to clean your lashes every day and especially after coming inside your home from cleaning in a dirty location like your garage, attic, or gardening outside. This simple step of washing your face and eyes can prevent a stye.

Eyelid Sprays or Sanitizers

Eyelid cleansers are more for cleaning the crusting and bacteria off your lids like soap. Eyelid sprays are for keeping the lids clean and killing skin bacteria around your lids. Many eyelid sprays are helpful in keeping your lashes clean from skin bacteria and preventing Demodex from recurring.

They all have hypochlorous acid of a low concentration ranging from 0.1–0.2% in them. Some brands include Heyedrate PRO by PRN, Oasis, Avenova, Acuicyn (prescription only), Theratears, and OCuSOFT Hypochlor. These are game changers if you have had numerous styes or chalazions over time and can help with regular dry eye too. I have patients who have recurrent styes, and once I put them on the eyelid sprays every night, they have not had a recurrence and don't have to worry about styes. These eyelid sprays can also help your dry eye and eye comfort.

Eyelid Lubricants

Another off-label but effective therapy for dry eye and blepharitis is using castor oil on your eyelashes (Sandford et al. al) along with Vaseline or coconut oil. If you are going to try this treatment, the castor oil needs to be cosmetic grade, organic, and hexane free. It is available on Amazon as well. It is not the version that is used for constipation. Pure castor oil can be sticky but is relatively safe for your eyes (I've used it myself). Sanford et al present the various properties that make it an effective treatment, including being anti-microbial and anti-inflammatory, and it smothers the Demodex mites, not allowing them to proliferate overnight. Vaseline works similarly when applied to the eyelid and up to the lash line and has been shown to be safe and effective even in babies. I have even seen significant eyelid inflammation with ocular rosacea calm down with the use of Vaseline. Many of my patients who are allergic to prescription medications for their blepharitis do well with these treatments even long term.

Warm Compresses vs. Cold Compresses

Warm compresses help soothe eyes that are fatigued; they help the oil flow out of your meibomian glands more effectively. I recommend using a wet washcloth or an eye mask to help hold heat on closed eyelids. You may need about 5–10 minutes of heat to support the oil glands and ensure the temperature is not too hot for your skin, or it may burn your skin. A wet washcloth will get cold in 1–2 minutes, so sometimes, an eye mask may be more effective. There are many eye masks on the market as well (Eye Eco DERM mask, Bruder mask, Tranquileyes, even electric masks which stay hot for some time), which will hold the temperature of the meibomian glands at the ideal temperature to help the oil glands flow better.

However, some patients may feel their eyes are worse with warm compresses. If allergies are a large factor in your dry eye, then cool compresses may be better for you, as heat can activate all of the allergy cells (mast cells, basophils, and eosinophils). If cool compresses are more soothing, you can use them. Cold compresses usually help to calm down allergic inflammation, so if cool compresses are better for you, you may need to focus more on anti-allergy treatments, including anti-allergy eye drops, oral pills, and nasal sprays. Please always listen to your body and what it tells you to do. Cold calms down allergic inflammation everywhere, even if you have a rash on your arm, and heat can make it worse, allowing the cells of your immune response to ramp up their histamine release and make everything worse. So, if your body says heat/warm compresses are making you worse, please stop and try cold compresses.

Amazing tip: Another tip is to use your eye drops cold. You can put artificial tears or anti-allergy drops in the fridge. It's like a cold shower for your eyes: refreshing and calming. The cold temperature can also help decrease the release of histamines from the immune cells that may be causing the allergic or inflammatory reaction.

PRESCRIPTION TREATMENTS

Nasal Spray for Dry Eye Called Tyrvaya

We already talked about anti-allergy nasal sprays. However, there's even a dry eye medication delivered as a nasal spray. It treats dry eye disease by stimulating the nasociliary nerve inside the nose with nasal spray aimed at the nerve and not into the back of the nose or sinuses. It is called Tyrvaya (varenicline 0.03 mg nasal spray). Some of my patients have given me great feedback that it can help their eyes feel normal within 1–2 weeks of use. If instilled incorrectly, it can cause burning inside your nose and sneezing. Don't worry, for most people the sneezing subsides and decreases after a few days of use. It is also a twice-daily medication; you cannot use it more. You cannot use it as needed, just like any other medication. Since it is relatively new, it may not have the best insurance coverage, but it is improving daily, and your doctor may have a sample for you to try if you're interested. My patients who have trouble instilling eye drops love this treatment as it helps their dry eye and they don't "waste" drops missing their eyes.

Antibiotic Ointments and Anti-Parasite Creams

If you have significant blepharitis from a skin infection like Staphylococcus bacteria, then using a prescription antibiotic ointment can help clear up the eyelid infection and help your dry eye symptoms. There are many types, including erythromycin (which is safe in children), bacitracin, neomycin, polymyxin, gentamycin, tobramycin, and sulfacetamide. You must make sure they are the "ophthalmic" version which is safe to get in your eyes and <u>not</u> the regular antibiotic cream you can buy over the counter. Another drop that has been used for blepharitis is azithromycin (the medicine in a Z-Pak but formulated as an eye drop), which can help and has been sold under the brand name Azasite and is also compounded by ImprimisRx pharmacy. I also mentioned ivermectin 1% earlier which is a cream I prescribe if I see Demodex mites living in your eyelashes. Ivermectin cream kills the mites, but they have a 2-week lifecycle, so you must use this cream for at least two life cycles or 4 weeks to get rid of mites. It is not safe to get in your eyes, so I tell patients to use the smallest amount possible and apply it to the base of the eyelashes. If it is getting in your eyes, you are using too much. This is an off-label use, so please talk to your doctor prior to using it to make sure it is safe for you.

Medicated Eye Drops

There are many prescription options for treating your dry eye disease if the above treatments do not help you enough. The most commonly known prescription eye drops are Restasis (0.05% cyclosporine), Cequa (0.09% cyclosporine), Xiidra (lifitegrast 5%), and Klarity-C (0.1% compounded cyclosporine by ImprimisRx). Depending on the FDA application and approval process, they have been given designations for helping many aspects of dry eye disease, such as treating the signs and/or symptoms of dry eye disease based on the study parameters. They are all anti-inflammatory medications and block the cells causing inflammation. Most of these cells live about 90 days, so it truly takes taking these medications 90 days of using them 2x per day for the medications to have full efficacy and help your dry eye disease. Many have been proven to start helping dry eye within 2–4 weeks, with both the signs and symptoms. There are differences in the side effects, including mild burning with instillation versus blurry vision for up to 5 minutes. Please talk to your eye doctor about these if you think you may be a candidate.

Please do not use them here and there (I hear this so commonly)! If you are doing this, you are truly using them as a lubricant, not as a medication to help your dry eye disease.

They are medications and have specific dosing guidelines for a reason, to help them effectively do the job you want them to do. If you use them when you feel dry, 1–2x every few days, they will not work as intended. If you did not give them a 90–100-day trial using them 2x per day (about 12 hours apart, then you cannot say they did not work. If you have too many side effects from them, then please talk to your eye doctor.

There are other medications that your doctor may use for severe dry eye disease, such as compounded cyclosporine 2% drops in oil for severe melting autoimmune corneal ulcers or medications like tacrolimus 0.03% eye drops or ointment (brand name Protopic at 0.03% or 0.1%) for immune suppression (which is not approved for use in the eye). I will not go into this any more than to mention it and let your doctor decide what is best for you.

An important tip for all medicated eye drops: Please make sure to close your eye for at least *30 seconds* after you instill drops to allow the medication to be absorbed into your eye. Sometimes I wonder if patients "fail" or don't respond to medications because they are just blinking them away instead of allowing proper absorption of the medication.

Cenergermin (Oxervate)

Cenergermin 0.002% (brand name Oxervate) is a promising prescription eye drop that can help patients with corneal nerve damage with neurotrophic keratitis. It was FDA-approved in 2018 and is a recombinant human nerve growth factor (rhNGF) medication. It is dosed at 6x per day for 8 weeks to help the damaged corneal nerves and severe dry eye disease. I have not used this medication for any patients yet as I've had great success with serum drops for these patients.

Regener-Eyes

Regener-Eyes is another option for some patients, which is officially over the counter but only sold through the company's website (see resources section) and with a doctor's recommendation. It is a proprietary formula of a placenta-derived product that has growth factors and nutrients that can help moderate to severe dry eye. The placenta is donated after a C-section delivery only and then tested to be safe, and a proprietary process extracts the nutrients. They have two formulas: the Lite, which does not have to be refrigerated, and the regular formula, which does need to be refrigerated. I do have a couple of patients who are on serum drops (next section) and use the Lite formula when they are traveling, so they don't have to worry about keeping serum drops cold. One does notice relief, and the other one doesn't. I don't have a lot of experience with this company yet.

Specialty Eye Drops – Autologous Serum Drops

If all else fails, it is time for autologous serum drops or blood drops, as some of my patients call them. These are drops made from your blood. Yes, I'm an eye doctor that draws blood in my office, and so does my staff. There are a few of us out there. We draw six tubes of tiger tops, and then my staff spins your blood down (in the centrifuge) and refrigerates them until the local compounding pharmacy picks the blood up, usually the same day or the next day. The pharmacy processes it based on my prescription for either 20% or 50% concentration of serum to BSS (balanced salt solution) and then puts it into bottles for you to use. Our local pharmacy (Rx3 pharmacy in Chester, VA) even delivers the serum drops to you on ice, or you can pick them up from the pharmacy. With six tubes of blood, they can usually get at least 12–15 bottles for you. All but one of the bottles need to stay frozen in the freezer, and those are good for two to six months generally. The one you are using should stay in the refrigerator, and that is good for 2 weeks unless you contaminate it, or you let it get too warm.

One important tip is to close your eyes for *3 full minutes* after instillation of the serum tears to help your eyes fully absorb your drops and not blink them away. Just like most eye drops where you should close your eyes for at least 30 seconds to 1 minute to let it fully absorb, except serum drops are longer. I've even had glaucoma patients who would blink their medications away, and this one simple tip of closing their eyes allowed their eyes to respond to their medications better, and their glaucoma was better controlled. I've had success treating severe dry eye patients with serum drops.

There was a study that helped me understand what we discussed earlier about "neuropathic dry eye" disease, which showed the neuromas on confocal microscopy. It also showed that over time, 4–12 months, with 4 times per day dosing with serum drops, patients improved in their pain, and dry eye, and the neuromas seemed improved/resolved as well. The corneal nerves were able to regrow to appear mostly normal on repeat confocal microscopy testing. There are wonderful growth factors and nutrients in our blood that we can harness to help heal our eyes. This concept is not new as people use serum for many other cosmetic procedures – if you have heard of PRP (platelet-rich plasma) being injected or micro-needled in the face for collagen building and facial rejuvenation and on the scalp for hair regrowth. Sometimes, I put patients on serum drops every 1–2 hours while awake to help heal their corneas. I also had a patient who used it inside of her soft contact lens, which helped her, similar to the fluid reservoir in a scleral lens (another specialty lens that can help some patients with corneal disease and dry eye disease). There is a national company called *Vital Tears* which also helps provide serum drops to those patients who don't have a local compounding pharmacy as we do here in Richmond, VA.

Autologous serum drops, even at 50% concentration, have been shown to be safe when used even long term (up to 4 years) without any complications (Hussain et al.). Serum drops could also help regrow corneal nerves that are affected during a LASIK procedure and help decrease the risk of dry eye afterward. A similar study showed cyclosporine 0.05% drops to be effective with a similar proposed mechanism of action (Kanellopoulos) postoperatively as well as preoperatively (Torricelli et al.).

Bandage Contact Lenses

Using contact lenses as a bandage can sometimes help dry eye disease and sometimes make it worse. It can help if the cornea is having trouble healing, as in severe damage, especially if there is a persistent scratch on the eye (persistent epithelial defect or PED), as it prevents the eyelid from touching the cornea and making things worse. Sometimes, bandage CLs are used in combination with serum drops, as mentioned above, and sometimes with amniotic membranes (fresh frozen preferred, but sometimes the dehydrated membranes, which act like collagen shields) can also help. Read the amniotic membrane section below. If the contact lens is the culprit of the corneal damage with lack of oxygen to the corneal epithelium, especially if the contact lens is too loose or too tight or overworn without a break (more than a normal workday of 8–10 hours) and it causes scratches on the cornea, damage to the limbal stem cells or the conjunctiva under the eyelids, then contact lens use can lead to a corneal ulcer or contact lens keratitis (inflammation from CL overwear). I saw a few cases of pingueculitis (inflammation of a pinguecula or yellow area on top of the sclera, usually next to the cornea in the horizontal meridian) with calcium deposits which I think may have become inflamed because of the patient's regular contact lens rubbing on the calcium and opening up the pinguecula or opening up on its own. Contact lenses are great, but sometimes they can cause the problem. Make sure you talk to your doctor about whether it is safe for you to wear contact lenses while undergoing dry eye treatment.

IN-OFFICE PROCEDURES

Punctal Plugs

If you do not have many tears, punctal plugs are a simple solution to help your dry eye. I do not use plugs in patients who have watering, as it can make their watering worse. They can also make you worse if you have a lot of inflammation on your ocular surface. Punctal plugs are either dissolvable or non-dissolvable. Many companies make punctal plugs. I describe them as little silicone stoppers which plug up your tear ducts, so more tears stay on the surface of your eyes and less drain away. They are easy to place in your tear ducts, take about less than 1–2 minutes at the most, and are done in the office. They are generally covered by insurance. They have some risks, including falling out or causing a tear duct infection. Even I had punctal plugs in my eyes for about 11 years until one day when I accidentally pulled them out while wiping something from the corner of my eyes. They are the only way I was able to wear contact lenses at my wedding (a simple request from my mother). If they cause a tear duct infection, we would have to remove them and treat you with antibiotics. They can also cause scar tissue to form in your tear ducts. At times, doctors use cautery to purposefully close the tear ducts permanently if you cannot tolerate plugs, but they do help your dry eye disease if there is minimal risk of watering.

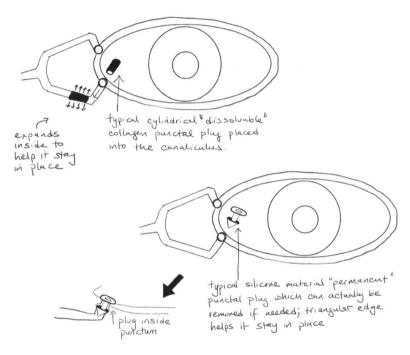

expands inside to help it stay in place.

typical cylindrical "dissolvable" collagen punctal plug placed into the canaliculus.

typical silicone material "permanent" punctal plug, which can actually be removed if needed; triangular edge helps it stay in place

plug inside punctum

Diagram #4

Intense Pulsed Light (IPL)

One of my favorite treatments for dry eye disease from meibomian gland dysfunction is IPL, or "intense pulsed light." It is a scattered light therapy that has been around for many decades for helping patients with rosacea and age spots. It was studied and proven to help dry eye disease within the last 15 years. IPL has become my go-to treatment if you are a candidate based on your skin type. I use the Lumenis M22 machine with the IPL handpiece. IPL has many benefits to your eyes and around the eyes. During the procedure, I numb the eyes with numbing eye drops and place laser-grade shields under your eyelids. Then I apply the IPL handpiece using clear ultrasound jelly to your face per the dry eye protocol developed by Dr. Toyos and additional treatment directly to the upper eyelids. After your first treatment, I also perform manual expression or squeeze the eyelids with a cotton-tipped applicator and try to get your meibomian glands flowing again. I always listen to you, and if it is too painful, we do a gentle expression. It will get everything flowing, so you may wake up the next day with crusty eyelashes from all the clogged oil flowing out. I do recommend that you use sunscreen in the area of treatment afterward for 2 weeks and use warm compresses 2–3x per day for the next 2–3 days.

What makes you a candidate? If I see poor oil secretions on the slit lamp exam or structural damage to your oil glands on your LipiScan test (imaging test for your meibomian glands), I will offer the procedure. There are risks, including sunburn (especially if you have been in the sun in the last 2 weeks in the area of treatment or a tanning bed or taking any medications or herbal supplements which may make you more prone to sunburns). There is a grading scale for skin types called the Fitzpatrick scale. IPL is unsafe for Fitzpatrick 5–6 skin types as it can cause darkening of your skin (hyperpigmentation).

How does it work? It helps so many parts of the eye. IPL can help photo-coagulate (close) the inflammatory blood vessels on the eyelid (telangiectasias), decreasing inflammation on the ocular surface and the meibomian glands. The heat also helps the oil glands flow better. The IPL energy also kills skin bacteria and Demodex mites (but not their eggs, as far as I can tell). IPL helps stimulate collagen building of the skin around the eye, and I've seen it help mild ectropion (where your eyelid is turning out away from your eye) to improve and help how well opposed the eyelid is to the eyeball. IPL helps stimulate the stem cells of the oil glands, allowing better oil production from the meibomian glands. IPL has also been shown to help with allergic conjunctivitis. When testing the glands on a LipiScan test, I have seen structural changes occur about 6–9 months after treatment, like longer glands. Luckily, I see functional changes with better oil flow, and patients feel better within 1–3 months after 1–3 treatments. I usually recommend that patients start with two treatments about 4 weeks apart and then see how they feel and how the meibomian glands produce oil on their next visit with the slit lamp exam. Depending on the starting level of damage, some patients may feel significant improvement for 6–12 months and then come in for a treatment or maintenance visit to help keep their meibomian glands functioning at their best. Omega-3s by mouth are also essential to help the meibomian glands function optimally.

LipiFlow

LipiFlow is an FDA-approved thermal pulsation device that heats your eyelids to a specific temperature and then applies calculated firm pressure on the upper and lower eyelids to help the oil flow out better. It can be used in patients who are not a candidate for IPL. I've had mixed reviews for the LipiFlow; some patients feel a huge difference for a while, and some only notice improvement for 2–4 weeks. Clinically after examining them, I can see a difference for some time. It is not my preferred therapy if you have meibomian gland disease as it may not help you with the structural changes as much as IPL. I have not seen any studies comparing the two modes of treating meibomian gland disease at this time. I have even had the LipiFlow done on myself, and I was underwhelmed by the results regarding how I felt. If patients are interested, I offer it to patients who are not candidates for IPL.

Meibomian Gland Probing

Dr. Steven Maskin in Florida started a micro-surgical procedure called meibomian gland probing in the office. He is able to demonstrate the breaking of scar tissue or fibrosis that builds up in the meibomian glands after years of chronic dysfunction to help stimulate the stem cells in the glands to help regrowth. After the probing procedure, he uses a micro-cannula to inject dexamethasone into the meibomian glands. He was so kind to train me for hours over Zoom during the COVID-19 pandemic, and his patients were also very kind to let me ask questions about the procedure. The results seem to last anywhere from 3–6 months until the procedure needs to be repeated, similar to the IPL and the LipiFlow procedures.

Amniotic Membrane

Many products on the market are derived from amniotic membranes. One of them that is FDA-approved for dry eye disease is Prokera (harvested by Biotissue). It is also FDA-approved for many other diagnoses like a severe corneal ulcer, keratitis, non-healed corneal abrasion (persistent epithelial defect), recurrent erosion syndrome, and many others. It is a cryopreserved amniotic membrane processed and attached to a silicone ring. Again, it is harvested after a healthy delivery via C-section and after testing the mom for any infectious disease. There are no abortions or other scenarios involved. Amniotic membrane transplantation is abbreviated as AMT. The doctor places the ring with the membrane on your eye, which typically dissolves in 3–7 days. I've had many patients with corneal erosions or melting corneal ulcers from rheumatoid arthritis who have improved significantly using the Prokera AMT.

I've also used Prokera in severe dry eye patients with significant corneal disease history and in patients with limbal stem cell deficiency. I know some doctors use it for mild dry eye, too (however, I do not). It can be expensive, although it is covered by insurance (sometimes needing a pre-authorization). There are a few versions of the Prokera, but most doctors use the *Prokera Slim* as the silicone ring is the most comfortable, and the thickness of the membrane is the same. Most other people cannot tell you have the Prokera on your eye, but it will blur your vision as it is a translucent but not transparent membrane you have to look through.

Other amniotic membranes on the market are dehydrated and not cryopreserved like the Prokera. They do have a role in corneal disease and dry eye disease. These are usually placed on the eye, and then a contact lens is used to cover the dried AMT, and these also dissolve in about 3–7 days. I've had success with one brand of this as well in the past. These don't have the biological properties found in the cryopreserved version, but they have the collagen and other dehydrated properties of the AMD.

In surgery with corneal melts, I have also used the cryopreserved membrane to fill the area of the corneal thinning/melt (which is more common in autoimmune diseases like rheumatoid arthritis) and then sutured on a layer on top of that. This is uncommon; I don't think most people will ever encounter such a situation.

Treatment for Conjunctivochalasis (CCH)

Sometimes, treating dry eye disease with the above-mentioned treatments resolves the symptoms of CCH. If it does not, there are surgical treatments for CCH, including cautery of the conjunctiva to shrink the extra conjunctiva in the office. This shrinking treatment can be done with a regular cautery or a specialized plasma pen like the one from Nuvissa (which can also be used for cosmetic procedures like tightening upper and lower eyelid skin). You can also have surgery in the operating room to remove the extra conjunctiva, usually in combination with placing an amniotic membrane in the area of resection to help build tighter adhesion of the tissue when it heals so the CCH does not recur. Dr. Periman has a cocktail called Laura's Lid Lifter (LLL) which can help lift the eyelid for up to 8 hours and reduce the folds in the redundant conjunctiva, thereby helping some patients with CCH. This cocktail is a mixture of Systane artificial tears, Upneeq (oxymetazoline 0.1%), and Lumify (brimonidine 0.025%)—note that this is not a usual treatment but could help some patients, and you will need to talk to your doctor if you want to try this or if it is appropriate for you.

ORAL MEDICATIONS

Doxycycline

Another treatment option for meibomian gland dysfunction causing dry eye disease is an oral medication called doxycycline. In dry eye disease, we typically use it at a low anti-inflammatory dose versus the total antibiotic dose unless indicated for an eyelid infection. The low dose of 40–50 mg of doxycycline for 2–4 weeks or longer can help decrease inflammation on both the ocular surface and the meibomian glands. The full dose of 100 mg 2x per day for 2 weeks is required for some patients depending on their level of eyelid inflammation. We know all antibiotics kill good healthy gut bacteria, and gut health is so important to overall health and eye health. I don't use this medication or other antibiotics unless I need to. However, I still use it occasionally and in patients with significant styes or chalazions, but not nearly as much as I used to 5–10 years ago.

Imidazoles Like Fluconazole

Interestingly, patients with seborrheic dermatitis (redness and peeling skin with inflammation and excess sebum/oil production) are thought to be linked to the fungus Malassezia spp. Treating the fungus with an anti-fungal like fluconazole can help the skin infection and chronic skin inflammation. Similarly, patients with seborrheic blepharitis, which is not Demodex, can also benefit from treatment with fluconazole. The treatment is usually 50 mg daily for 2–4 weeks, however, this dose is not available in the USA. Another anti-fungal drug that can be used for skin infections is terbinafine, but this has not been studied for blepharitis. As with all medications, talk to your doctor, check for drug interactions, and make sure the medication is right for you and your body. I have not tried these in my patients.

Acupuncture

Believe it or not, acupuncture has been studied for dry eye and has been used for decades (probably centuries) for dry eye disease as well as many other diseases. Acupuncture uses the ancient Eastern art of tapping into pressure points using tiny needles throughout our body which can help relieve many ailments including dry eye disease. It is possible to have some relief with mild massage as well. Real acupuncture should be done by a licensed acupuncture professional/specialist or a certified (doctor or dentist also trained in acupuncture) acupuncture specialist. There are 127 results that show up on PubMed when searching dry eye and acupuncture (including human and animal studies). There are human studies showing acupuncture improves tear break-up time, Schirmer's and OSDI scores (Prinz et al.). There's another review article looking at 19 clinical trials that showed similar results with improvement of dry eye disease with treatments 1–2 times per week for at least a month (Kim et al.) and a few other review articles with similar results and even some in subgroups like dry eye after cataract surgery, after refractive surgery, and in diabetes. The mechanism of action could be anti-inflammatory as it was shown to decrease inflammatory markers (IL-6 and TNF-α) in the tear film (Lin et al). Ask your doctor if acupuncture could be useful for you and find a qualified specialist.

SOME INTERESTING "EYE PAIN" CASE REPORTS

Serum drops can also help with recurrent erosion syndrome. Years ago, I had one patient with recurrent erosions and continuous eye pain despite good clinical and surgical treatment, including PTK (phototherapeutic keratectomy) multiple times by another doctor, who finally resolved after treatment with serum drops for 6–12 months. She had common immune variable deficiency (CVID), which may have contributed to her eye condition as well.

I had another patient who had bilateral corneal transplants years ago, and then one eye became painful. His local eye doctor treated him with Prokera (we discussed this in the amniotic membrane section) without relief. He wanted to take his "eyes out" (that's how severe his pain was) or get another transplant. He had recurrent corneal erosions and opened up areas of his epithelium many times, which I could see on his first visit. I debrided his cornea and performed a diamond burr polish to his basement membrane to reset his corneal epithelial attachments. I started him on serum drops and oral doxycycline at 50 mg daily for 3–6 months, and with treatment, I was able to get him pain-free within 1–2 weeks and prevented him from ever having another erosion and healing his eyes. He did not need another corneal transplant.

I had another patient who had a corneal abrasion from a Christmas card scratching her eye and had recurrent erosions for six months before seeing me. At presentation, I debrided her irregular cornea and later performed PTK to get her pain-free and reset her corneal epithelium. She did not use a serum but did use doxycycline and a bandage contact lens under my close supervision for months until she was not scared to take it off. She is doing great without another episode of erosion many years later.

Another patient referred for severe dry eyes was on three glaucoma eye drops and had red irritated eyes with scar tissue developing indicating pseudopemphigoid and toxicity from the preservatives in his eye drops. He was living with severely irritated eyes and not a great quality of life. After a careful review of his records and glaucoma testing and coordination with his glaucoma specialist, we stopped all his medications and let his eyes breathe, which resolved his symptoms, along with oral omega-3s. We needed to treat his mild glaucoma with alternative methods (laser) that would not make his conjunctiva continue scarring further. He did not need any other dry eye treatment. Sometimes, we need to step back and re-evaluate all the treatments a patient is on and stop them all, which can ultimately help the patient more than additional medications.

All of these patients have been doing well for some time now. If you have dry eyes, whether typical or atypical, it's important to see a dry eye specialist—who is a cornea specialist and ophthalmologist like me—to get the right diagnosis and treatment.

5

LIFESTYLE MEDICINE AND THE SIX PILLARS OF HEALTH

L ifestyle Medicine is a relatively new field of medicine with evidence-based medicine with six pillars of health which apply to eyes and eye diseases. I became interested in the field and took the test to become board-certified in 2020. The six pillars of health are whole-food, plant-based nutrition/diet, physical activity, stress management, avoidance of risky substances (like tobacco/alcohol/drugs), restorative sleep, and social connection.

NUTRITION

Nutrition has a huge role in our bodies and the development of chronic diseases. Changing our nutrition can help prevent and reverse chronic diseases, including in the eyes. I talk to patients about anti-inflammatory diets for dry eye disease as well. An anti-inflammatory diet includes adding food that is anti-inflammatory and avoiding food that is pro-inflammatory. We talked about adding omega-3s already, which are anti-inflammatory. Other food/supplements which are known to be anti-inflammatory include berries, turmeric (curcumin with bioperine)—read more on my blog about turmeric—food with high fiber like fruits and vegetables, and phytochemicals as found in nuts, whole grains, and green leafy vegetables (like Dr. Caldwell Esselstyn's favorites of kale, spinach, Swiss chard, arugula, beet greens, beets, bok choy, collard greens, mustard greens, turnip greens, napa cabbage, brussels sprouts, broccoli, cauliflower, cilantro, parsley, and asparagus). Many studies looking at Mediterranean diets along with various levels and forms of omega-3s have shown that a healthy diet with fresh food, low fat, and high omega-3 helps dry eye disease. Turmeric (curcumin with bioperine) can be beneficial for dry eye disease at 500 mg per day, but it can cause you to be more sensitive to sunburns, so be careful.

Removing pro-inflammatory food is also important. For example, processed food, like the preservatives in cheese curl snacks, is not nutritious and can be pro-inflammatory. Processed meat and high amounts of dairy are also pro-inflammatory. The World Health Organization (WHO) has labeled processed meat as a carcinogen and linked it to colon cancer. Dairy has also been shown to have a high association with various cancers. Both processed meat and dairy have been linked to strokes and heart attacks. Removing them may also help your dry eye disease. I've had numerous patients with severe eye pain, which was ignored but really due to sinus disease, and eliminating dairy from their diets (along with antibiotics) helped their pain. One patient with thyroid disease and prior sinus surgery who still had eye pain listened and eliminated dairy in her diet and was finally pain-free after one year of struggling.

Another fact that supports inflammation being the main cause of dry eye disease—whether the inflammation is on the eyelids in the meibomian glands or on the ocular surface with the conjunctiva and goblet cells—is that all of our dry eye medications (cyclosporine 0.05% or 0.09% or lifitegrast 5%) block the inflammatory cells on the ocular surface to help dry eye. If we can help this process by changing our diet as well, why not help ourselves?

I'm constantly telling my patients to take their multivitamins in addition to omega-3s. Yes, with an ideal diet, we would not need vitamins. But we don't all have ideal diets. If you have any gut problems, you may not be absorbing all the nutrients you're eating, even with the ideal diet of leafy green vegetables, fiber, and fresh fruits and vegetables. Looking at some scientific studies, the Blue Mountains Eye Study showed many examples of food affecting the eyes, although not specifically dry eyes, including flavonoid-rich food (like leafy vegetables) helping decrease mortality even if you had other risk factors for poor health (like smoking, drinking, lack of exercise) (Croft et al.). Another subset showed "Intakes of a broad range of micro- and macro-nutrients were significantly and independently associated with reduced odds of experiencing dry eye symptoms" (Guo et al.). These included B12, Vitamin C, B1, polyunsaturated fats, and calcium. I won't cover all the numerous studies showing lifestyle changes that affect dry eye disease. But please listen to common sense and what your mother may have told you and eat 5–7 servings of fruits and vegetables, 25 grams of fiber, and a full rainbow color of food to help your dry eye too. The Blue Mountains Eye Study with 422 results published on PubMed showed us many effects of diet on various parts of the eye, including cataracts and glaucoma.

GLUTEN

Gluten is also pro-inflammatory. I have been gluten-free for about 5–6 years now, and my dry eye is definitely better without gluten. Without getting too much into my medical history, being gluten-free has also helped my fertility, dizziness, nausea, and stomach issues. I have a patient with Celiac disease who has eye irritation/flare-ups every time she accidentally eats gluten. I have many other patients with iritis (inflammation of the iris) who have a flare-up of their intraocular inflammation when they eat gluten. Ankylosing spondylitis (HLA-B27 positive) is another systemic autoimmune inflammatory condition that can cause iritis and is known to flare up with gluten intake. One study showed a

14.7% risk of Celiac disease if the patient has Sjogren's disease (Iltanen et al.). Many autoimmune diseases run together as the patient's baseline level of inflammation is high in their whole body.

SYSTEMIC AUTOIMMUNE INFLAMMATION

Glover et al. does a great job reviewing ocular manifestations in autoimmune disease and has a striking table where keratoconjunctivitis sicca (another name for dry eye disease) is checked off as occurring in almost every single autoimmune disorder of the body. Dry eye is found in 10–35% of rheumatoid arthritis patients, 18.75% of psoriasis patients, 64% of systemic sclerosis patients, up to 21% of myasthenia gravis patients, and up to 85% in thyroid-associated eye disease (Glover et al.). "1 in 3 patients with Sjogren's syndrome shows ocular manifestations, with 13% of this being sight-threatening. Like rheumatoid arthritis, dry eye disease is the most common ocular manifestation. Acting as a precursor, 1 in 10 American patients over the age of 50 diagnosed with dry eye disease ultimately have underlying Sjogren's syndrome" (Glover et al.). This article also highlights that women tend to get more autoimmune diseases overall and constitute up to 85% of all patients with autoimmune diseases and goes into more detail about the genetic reasons for the disease prevalence and severity differences we see in both genders. This data is so powerful and shows how common inflammation is as the cause of dry eye disease throughout the whole body. Treatment with systemic medications can help dry eye but a few can make it worse, so make sure to talk to your doctor about your medications as well.

SUGAR IS INFLAMMATORY

We are learning more and more about how sugar can cause inflammation. Dr. Maskin's research has shown that the meibomian glands are more dysfunctional with high blood sugar and in diabetic patients, which can lead to more dry eye disease and worse MGD. Another study showed worsening dry eye with worsening diabetic retinopathy (amount of bleeding in your retina from diabetes) but not duration of diabetes (Nadeem et al.). An older study showed a striking statistic: 52.8% of diabetic patients had dry eye disease compared to 9.3% of control patients with higher rates of dry eye with higher HbA1c levels (Seifart et al.). Another large study showed diabetic patients use almost double the amount of lubrication (20.6 vs 13.8%) compared to non-diabetics and more when their HbA1c was higher (Kaiserman et al.). We know diabetic patients have nerve damage which can lead to poorly healing ulcers in their feet (peripheral neuropathy). Perhaps there is also some nerve damage in the cornea leading to worsening dry eye disease too and a dysfunctional feedback loop leading to worse dry eyes. If your eyes are not getting better, consider going to see your PCP and check your blood sugar levels. Listen to your body and give up gluten and sugar if it leads to happier eyes and healthier bodies.

HYDRATION

Hydration with adequate water intake is also important for treating dry eye disease. How can you expect to have hydrated eyes if you are not giving your body the proper amount of water daily? Our bodies are about 60–70% water; we need water to live. You should drink about 8–12 cups of water per day and maybe more if you are engaging in heavy exercise during the day or live in extreme climate conditions. Systemic dehydration has also been shown to lower tear osmolarity tests (which we discussed earlier is a test used by some doctors to show your level of dry eyes) and correlated with dry eye disease (Walsh et al.). So drinking more water can give you more tears and a healthier concentration of tears.

POLYPHARMACY

Polypharmacy is a term that means many systemic medications can cause significant additive side effects together. Please ask your primary care doctor and ophthalmologist if any other medications could worsen your dry eye disease. We've earlier discussed BAK, a preservative in most eye drops, and taking multiple medications like glaucoma drops and tear drops can cause ocular toxicity. Systemic medications, especially those with a decongestant (anything ending in -D like Claritin-D or Allegra-D), can cause worsening dry eye disease. Other systemic medications can be causing the problems. Not a large study, but one showed more dry eye if you were on a statin; however, no link to dry eye if you had high cholesterol vs. not (Ooi et al.). If you are not getting better, talk to your primary care doctor (PCP) about what systemic medications you are taking, which could worsen your dry eye disease. That reminds me of one patient who had intermittent blurry vision, and her eyes looked normal, including her angles, but I sent her back to her PCP, and her PCP figured out one of her irritable bowel disease drugs was causing her blurry vision, and it resolved after the patient stopped the offending drug. It was not due to dry eye disease or any other ocular cause.

PHYSICAL EXERCISE, STRESS MANAGEMENT, SOCIAL CONNECTION

Physical exercise, stress management, and social connection (which also helps in stress management) all help *decrease inflammation* in your body and can help dry eye disease as well. A study on office workers showed that a 10-week exercise program helped dry eye symptoms (Sano et al.). We know exercise decreases inflammation in our bodies, so that could be the mechanism of action. Another study showed similar improvement in dry eye symptoms (not signs) after two months of lifestyle changes, including diet modification, physical activity, and positive thinking (Kawashima et al.). Although stress management and social connection have not been studied specifically for dry eye, there is evidence that each factor, including sleep, is associated with significant aqueous deficiency and evaporative dry eye disease (Wolffsohn et al.).

RESTORATIVE SLEEP

We already talked about some sleep modifications which can help if you are sleeping with a CPAP mask or if you are sleeping on your face inducing floppy eyelid syndrome. Another important tip for sleep is to make sure you turn off your electronic devices at least 30 minutes (ideally 1 hour) before bedtime and help your body unwind after a long day. If you watch TV or shows on your tablet until you fall asleep, you may not have proper eyelid closure, which in turn can cause your eyes to dry out. I have had patients who slept poorly, either from sleeping too late or sleeping with some alcohol on board and wake up with corneal abrasions because they slept with their eyes open. If you want to learn more, one of my favorite books on sleep is called *The Promise of Sleep* by Dr. William Dement (who discovered REM sleep).

PREGNANCY AND HORMONES

Interestingly, my dry eye symptoms were much better during pregnancy and worse with breastfeeding. Some studies have observations with worsening dry eye symptoms in pregnancy. Another article points out that pregnancy decreases parts of the mother's immune system to protect the fetus, so certain autoimmune diseases could get better while others get worse (Glover et al.). Many of the dry eye medications available are safe to use in pregnancy if your symptoms indicate they are necessary. Diet can definitely affect hormones; one case report showed a reversal of ovarian failure with an elimination diet (removing gluten, meat, dairy, sugar, nightshade vegetables, and citrus) over 4 months (Feuerstein). Even my personal increased fertility with a gluten-free and vegan diet lends support to the regulation of hormones over a short 3–4 months time period.

MENOPAUSE

One study I saw showed that women have a higher incidence of dry eye disease, especially after menopause, without any estrogen replacement, and lower rates if they are on hormone replacement therapy (HRT) (Versura et al.). However, the Women's Health Study of over 25,000 patients showed an increased risk of dry eye disease using HRT with an odds ratio of 1.69x risk with estrogen alone and 1.29x risk with estrogen and progesterone compared to no HRT (Liesegang, TJ). There are risks to HRT, so I recommend listening to your body and talking to your PCP and gynecologist if you feel menopause or HRT are helping or harming your body.

AVOIDANCE OF RISKY SUBSTANCES

You can imagine exposure to smoke from smoking cigarettes can dry and irritate your eyes. Smoking and vaping can expose your eyes to the chemicals in the smoke, which can be a local irritant to your eyes. Smoking is also known to induce free radicals and be pro-inflammatory, making dry eye worse. Smoking can also delay corneal healing and cause progression of Fuchs' endothelial corneal dystrophy (Nita et al.). Smoking has also been known to exacerbate thyroid eye disease in patients with thyroid problems and cause inflammation, redness, and proptosis, and can also cause secondary worsening dry eye disease. Some large meta-analyses have failed to prove a causal effect, but common sense can tell you if your eyes feel worse when smoking or when you are around smoke, you need to avoid smoking or being around smoke vapors. Listen to your body and what it's trying to tell you. Some other meta-analyses showed a 50% higher risk of dry eye disease if you were a smoker or former smoker (Acar et al., Xu et al.).

Drinking alcohol can cause dehydration which can lead to dry eye (Magno et al.). Alcohol use is associated with dry eye disease, especially in women. A meta-analysis showed a 15% higher risk of dry eye for patients with alcohol consumption, even when accounting for smoking, hypertension, diabetes, and thyroid disease (You et al.). You et al. also discuss that alcohol has been noted to be present in the tear film, which can disrupt the tear film structure on the ocular surface and allow more inflammatory cytokines to be present on the ocular surface. This discussion reminds us that chronic alcoholism can cause vitamin A deficiency which is a known cause of severe dry eye disease. Alcohol can also not only cause peripheral neuropathy or nerve damage in the hands and feet but also in the corneal nerves and can disrupt the feedback loop of the tear film and cornea.

Again, this section on Lifestyle Medicine and dry eye disease is not meant to be a research paper-level analysis but a broad overview of how many factors can be associated with dry eye disease. If you suffer from dry eye disease, please also look at your overall health, nutrition, physical exercise, stress levels, sleep, smoking and alcohol use, and overall social network and positive connectedness with each other and nature.

CONCLUSION

I hope you found this book straightforward and helpful in helping to tackle your dry eye disease and giving you actionable steps to help yourself and be able to talk to your eye doctor to get you the help you need. As mentioned before, my goal is to normalize and optimize the ocular surface and treat your dry eyes so you don't think about them all the time, and they return to being a normal part of your body. Again, dry eye disease is a chronic condition and we may never be able to eliminate dry eye disease. However, if we can get you living a normal life without thinking about your eyes all the time, I think we are achieving success. I'm a minimalist. I will treat you and get you better but then try to get you off most medications except omega-3s. Check out the resources section to learn more. Check out my website for more information as well. You can also contact me for an educational consultation through my office if out of Virginia or a telemedicine consultation if you are located in Virginia.

Please leave a review: If you found this book helpful, *please leave a 5-star rating and a review on Amazon* and the platform you purchased this book to help spread the information and help more people with their dry eye disease. Please share this book with your family and friends who would benefit from reading it.

Thank you for taking the time to read, and I hope you find significant relief from your dry eyes with the tips in this book or at least directions on how to get help.

There is relief from dry eye disease! See your eye doctor for help if you still have symptoms of dry eye disease, get the comfort you deserve, and get back to your life.

RESOURCES

EYEWIKI

An excellent website for all things related to the eye is https://eyewiki.org—it is like Wikipedia but focuses on eye conditions. It is written and run by the American Academy of Ophthalmology, so you know you are getting an expert's information. Please ask your eye doctor to explain if the information is too detailed. Also, please always ask for help and do not attempt to treat yourself when you do not know the correct diagnosis.

Some great EyeWiki pages about dry eye and related conditions are:

Dry Eye Syndrome - EyeWiki. (2022, October 9). https://eyewiki.org/Dry_Eye_Syndrome.

Diagnostic Testing for Dry Eye - EyeWiki. (2022, October 29). https://eyewiki.org/Diagnostic_Testing_for_Dry_Eye.

Conjunctivochalasis - EyeWiki. (n.d.). *https://eyewiki.aao.org/Conjunctivochalasis.*

Recurrent Corneal Erosion - EyeWiki. (2022, July 23). https://eyewiki.org/Recurrent_Corneal_Erosion.

Thyroid Eye Disease - EyeWiki. (2023, January 11). https://eyewiki.org/Thyroid_Eye_Disease.

Exposure Keratopathy - EyeWiki. (2023, February 5). https://eyewiki.org/Exposure_Keratopathy.

Facial Nerve Palsy - EyeWiki. (2023, January 2). https://eyewiki.org/Facial_Nerve_Palsy.

Floppy Eyelid Syndrome - EyeWiki. (2022, September 23). https://eyewiki.org/Floppy_Eyelid_Syndrome.

Ophthalmologic Manifestations of Obstructive Sleep Apnea - EyeWiki. (2021, April 19). https://eyewiki.org/Ophthalmologic_Manifestations_of_Obstructive_Sleep_Apnea.

Mask Associated Dry Eye (MADE) - EyeWiki. (2022, April 6). https://eyewiki.org/Mask_Associated_Dry_Eye_(MADE).

Dry Eye in Sjogren's Syndrome - EyeWiki. (2022, September 11). https://eyewiki.org/Dry_Eye_in_Sjogren's_Syndrome.

Salzmann Nodular Degeneration - EyeWiki. (2022, September 11). https://eyewiki.org/Salzmann_Nodular_Degeneration.

Autologous and Allogenic Serum Tears - EyeWiki. (2022, December 7). https://eyewiki.org/Autologous_and_Allogenic_Serum_Tears.

Meibomian Gland Dysfunction (MGD) - EyeWiki. (2022, September 3). https://eyewiki.org/Meibomian_Gland_Dysfunction_(MGD).

Computer Vision Syndrome (Digital Eye Strain) - EyeWiki. (2022, April 6). https://eyewiki.org/Computer_Vision_Syndrome_(Digital_Eye_Strain).

Intense Pulsed Light (IPL) Therapy - EyeWiki. (2022, September 11). https://eyewiki.org/Intense_Pulsed_Light_(IPL)_Therapy.

OTHER REFERENCES

Eye Drops | AAAAI. (n.d.). https://www.aaaai.org/tools-for-the-public/drug-guide/eye-drops.

How Xiidra Works | Xiidra® (lifitegrast ophthalmic solution). (n.d.). https://www.xiidra.com/what-is-xiidra.

CEQUA® for Chronic Dry Eye | Patient Information. (n.d.). https://www.cequa.com/.

RESTASIS® Eye Drops for Chronic Dry Eye | RESTASIS®. (n.d.). https://www.restasis.com/.

Tyrvaya. (n.d.). https://www.tyrvaya.com/.

Home - OXERVATE® (cenegermin-bkbj). (2022b, July 28). OXERVATE® (Cenegermin-bkbj). https://oxervate.com/.

Maskin, S. Dry Eye, and Cornea Treatment Center. Retrieved February 25, 2023, from https://drmaskin.com/.

Serum Drops Made Simple. (n.d.). Vital Tears. https://vitaltears.org/.

The power of science, in the ease of an eye drop TM. (n.d.). Regener-Eyes Ophthalmic Solution. https://www.regenereyes.com/.

Prokera® Biologic Corneal Bandage. (2023, February 15). BioTissue. https://biotissue.com/products/ocular/prokera/.

Dement, W. C., & Vaughan, C. (2000). *The Promise of Sleep: A Pioneer in Sleep Medicine Explores the Vital Connection Between Health, Happiness, and a Good Night's Sleep.* Dell.

Fish and Omega-3 Fatty Acids. (2022, July 20). www.heart.org. https://www.

heart.org/en/healthy-living/healthy-eating/eat-smart/fats/fish-and-omega-3-fatty-acids.

Link, M. R. S. (2017, July 17). *The 7 Best Plant Sources of Omega-3 Fatty Acids.* Healthline. https://www.healthline.com/nutrition/7-plant-sources-of-omega-3s.

CITATIONS

Acar, D. E., Acar, U., Tunay, Z. Ö., Ozdemir, O., & Germen, H. (2017). The effects of smoking on dry eye parameters in healthy women. *Cutaneous and Ocular Toxicology, 36*(1), 1–4. https://doi.org/10.3109/15569527.2015.1136828.

Chen, H., Chen, A., Wang, S., Zou, M., Young, C. M., Zheng, D., & Jin, G. (2022). Association Between Migraine and Dry Eye: A Systematic Review and Metaanalysis. *Cornea, 41*(6), 740–745. https://doi.org/10.1097/ico.0000000000002851.

Croft, K. D., Lewis, J. R., Blekkenhorst, L. C., Bondonno, C. P., Shin, J. H., Woodman, R. J., Wong, G., Lim, W. H., Gopinath, B., Flood, V. M., Russell, J., Mitchell, P., & Hodgson, J. M. (2020). Association of flavonoids and flavonoid-rich foods with all-cause mortality: The Blue Mountains Eye Study. *Clinical Nutrition, 39*(1), 141–150. https://doi.org/10.1016/j.clnu.2019.01.004.

Feuerstein, J. (2010). Reversal of Premature Ovarian Failure in a Patient with Sjögren Syndrome Using an Elimination Diet Protocol. *Journal of Alternative and Complementary Medicine, 16*(7), 807–809. https://doi.org/10.1089/acm.2010.0022.

Glover, K., Mishra, D., & Singh, T. R. R. (2021). Epidemiology of Ocular Manifestations in Autoimmune Disease. *Frontiers in Immunology, 12.* https://doi.org/10.3389/fimmu.2021.744396.

Guo, B., Gopinath, B., Watson, S., Burlutsky, G., Mitchell, P., & Ooi, K. (2023). Associations between intake of dietary micro- and macro-nutrients with Dry eye syndrome. *Clinical Nutrition ESPEN, 54,* 258–263. https://doi.org/10.1016/j.clnesp.2023.01.019.

Hussain, M., Shtein, R. M., Sugar, A., Soong, H. K., Woodward, M. A., DeLoss, K. S., & Mian, S. I. (2014). Long-term Use of Autologous Serum 50% Eye

Drops for the Treatment of Dry Eye Disease. *Cornea, 33*(12), 1245–1251.https://doi.org/10.1097/ico.0000000000000271.

Iltanen, S., Collin, P., Korpela, M., Holm, K., Partanen, J., Polvi, A., & Mäki, M. (1999). Celiac Disease and Markers of Celiac Disease Latency in Patients With Primary Sjögren's Syndrome. *The American Journal of Gastroenterology, 94*(4), 1042–1046. https://doi.org/10.1111/j.1572-0241. 1999.01011.x.

Jones, L., Downie, L. E., Korb, D. R., Benitez-Del-Castillo, J. M., Dana, R., Deng, S. X., Dong, P. N., Geerling, G., Hida, R. Y., Liu, Y., Seo, K. Y., Tauber, J., Wakamatsu, T. H., Xu, J., Wolffsohn, J. S., & Craig, J. P. (2017). TFOS DEWS II Management and Therapy Report. *Ocular Surface, 15*(3), 575–628. https://doi.org/10.1016/j.jtos.2017.05.006.

Kaiserman, I., Kaiserman, N., Nakar, S., & Vinker, S. (2005). Dry eye in diabetic patients. *American Journal of Ophthalmology, 139*(3), 498–503. https://doi.org/10.1016/j.ajo.2004.10.022.

Kanellopoulos, A. J. (2019). Incidence and management of symptomatic dry eye related to LASIK for myopia, with topical cyclosporine A. *Clinical Ophthalmology, Volume 13*, 545–552. https://doi.org/10.2147/opth. s188521.

Kawashima, M., Sano, K., Takechi, S., & Tsubota, K. (2018). Impact of lifestyle intervention on dry eye disease in office workers: a randomized controlled trial. *Journal of Occupational Health, 60*(4), 281–288. https://doi. org/10.1539/joh.2017-0191-oa.

Kim, B., Kim, M., Kang, H., & Nam, H. (2018). Optimizing acupuncture treatment for dry eye syndrome: a systematic review. *BMC Complementary and Alternative Medicine, 18*(1). https://doi.org/10.1186/s12906-018-2202-0.

Koo, H. C., Kim, T. Y., Kim, K. H., Wee, S. H., Chun, Y. S., & Kim, J. N. (2012). Ocular Surface Discomfort and *Demodex*: Effect of Tea Tree Oil Eyelid Scrub in *Demodex* Blepharitis. *Journal of Korean Medical Science, 27*(12), 1574. https://doi.org/10.3346/jkms.2012.27.12.1574.

Liesegang, T. J. (2002). Hormone replacement therapy and dry eye syndrome. Schaumberg DA,∗∗Division of Preventive Medicine, Brigham and Women's Hospital, Harvard Medical School, 900 Commonwealth Ave E, Boston, MA 02215. USA E-mail: schaumberg@rics.bwh.harvard.edu Buring JE, Sullivan DA, Dana MR. JAMA 2001;286:2114–2119. *American*

Journal of Ophthalmology, 133(3), 435–436. https://doi.org/10.1016/s0002-9394(02)01368-5.

Lin, Z., Yu, D., Zhao, J., Shi, H., Zhang, Z., Zhao, L., & Ju, P. (2022). [Effect of acupuncture on dry eye and tear inflammatory factors]. *PubMed, 42*(12), 1379–1383. https://doi.org/10.13703/j.0255-2930.20220318-0001.

Magno, M. S., Daniel, T., Morthen, M. K., Snieder, H., Jansonius, N. M., Utheim, T. P., Hammond, C. J., & Vehof, J. (2021). The relationship between alcohol consumption and dry eye. *Ocular Surface, 21,* 87–95. https://doi.org/10.1016/j.jtos.2021.05.005.

Miljanovic, B., Trivedi, K. A., Dana, R., Gilbard, J. P., Buring, J. E., & Schaumberg, D. A. (2005). Relation between dietary n–3 and n–6 fatty acids and clinically diagnosed dry eye syndrome in women. *The American Journal of Clinical Nutrition,* 82(4), 887–893. *https://doi.org/10.1093/ajcn/82.4.887.*

Nadeem, H., Malik, T. G., Mazhar, A., & Ali, A. (2020). Association of Dry Eye Disease with Diabetic Retinopathy. *JCPSP. Journal of the College of Physicians & Surgeons Pakistan, 30*(05), 493–497. https://doi.org/10.29271/jcpsp.2020.05.493.

Nita, M., & Grzybowski, A. (2017). Smoking and Eye Pathologies. A Systemic Review. Part I. Anterior Eye Segment Pathologies. *Current Pharmaceutical Design,* 23(4), 629–638. https://doi.org/10.2174/1381612822666161129152041.

Ooi, K. G., Lee, M. J., Burlutsky, G., Gopinath, B., Mitchell, P., & Watson, S. L. (2019). Association of dyslipidaemia and oral statin use, and dry eye disease symptoms in the Blue Mountains Eye Study. *Clinical and Experimental Ophthalmology, 47*(2), 187–192. https://doi.org/10.1111/ceo.13388.

Prinz, J., Maffulli, N., Fuest, M., Walter, P., Hildebrand, F., & Migliorini, F. (2022). Acupuncture for the management of dry eye disease. *Frontiers of Medicine, 16*(6), 975–983. https://doi.org/10.1007/s11684-022-0923-4.

Rege, A., Kulkarni, V. P., Puthran, N., & Khandgave, T. P. (2013). A Clinical Study of Subtype-based Prevalence of Dry Eye. *Journal of Clinical and Diagnostic Research.* https://doi.org/10.7860/jcdr/2013/6089.3472.

Sandford, E. C., Muntz, A., & Craig, J. P. (2021). Therapeutic potential of castor oil in managing blepharitis, meibomian gland dysfunction and dry eye. *Clinical and Experimental Optometry, 104*(3), 315–322. https://doi.org/ 10.1111/cxo.13148.

Sano, K., Kawashima, M., Takechi, S., Mimura, M., & Tsubota, K. (2018). Exercise program improved subjective dry eye symptoms for office workers. *Clinical Ophthalmology, Volume 12*, 307–311. https://doi.org/10.2147/ opth.s149986.

Savla, K., Le, J. T., & Pucker, A. D. (2020). Tea tree oil for Demodex blepharitis. *The Cochrane Library, 2022*(1). https://doi.org/10.1002/14651858.cd013333.pub2.

Seifart U, Strempel I. Trockenes Auge und Diabetes mellitus [The dry eye and diabetes mellitus]. Ophthalmologe. 1994 Apr;91(2):235-9. German. PMID: 8012143.

Suwal, A., Hao, J., Zhou, D., Liu, X., Suwal, R., & Lu, C. (2020). Use of Intense Pulsed Light to Mitigate Meibomian Gland Dysfunction for Dry Eye Disease. *International Journal of Medical Sciences, 17*(10), 1385–1392. https://doi.org/10.7150/ijms.44288.

Tavassoli, S., Wong, N. D., & Chan, E. (2021). Ocular manifestations of rosacea: A clinical review. *Clinical and Experimental Ophthalmology, 49*(2), 104–117. https://doi.org/10.1111/ceo.13900.

Torricelli, A. A., Santhiago, M. R., & Wilson, S. E. (2014). Topical Cyclosporine A Treatment in Corneal Refractive Surgery and Patients With Dry Eye. *Journal of Refractive Surgery, 30*(8), 558–564. https://doi.org/10.3928/ 1081597x-20140711-09.

Versura, P., & Campos, E. C. (2005). Menopause and dry eye. A possible relationship. *Gynecological Endocrinology, 20*(5), 289–298. https://doi.org/10. 1080/09513590400027257.

Walsh, N. P., Fortes, M. B., Raymond-Barker, P., Bishop, C., Owen, J. A., Tye, E., Esmaeelpour, M., Purslow, C., & Elghenzai, S. (2012). Is Whole-Body Hydration an Important Consideration in Dry Eye? *Investigative Ophthalmology & Visual Science, 53*(10), 6622. https://doi.org/10.1167/iovs. 12-10175.

Wolffsohn, J. S., Wang, M., Vidal-Rohr, M., Menduni, F., Dhallu, S., Ipek, T., Acar, D., Recchioni, A., Kingsnorth, A., & Craig, J. P. (2021). Demographic and lifestyle risk factors of dry eye disease subtypes: A cross-sectional study. *Ocular Surface, 21*, 58–63. https://doi.org/10.1016/j.jtos.2021. 05.001.

Xu, L., Zhang, W., Zhu, X., Suo, T., Fan, X., & Fu, Y. (2016). Smoking and the risk of dry eye: a Meta-analysis. *International Journal of Ophthalmology.* https://doi.org/10.18240/ijo.2016.10.19.

Yang, W., Luo, Y., Wu, S., Niu, X., Yan, Y., Qiao, C., Ming, W., Zhang, Y., Wang, H., Chen, D., Qi, M., Ke, L., Wang, Y., Li, L., Li, S., & Zeng, Q. (2021). Estimated Annual Economic Burden of Dry Eye Disease Based on a Multi-Center Analysis in China: A Retrospective Study. *Frontiers in Medicine, 8.* https://doi.org/10.3389/fmed.2021.771352.

Yu, J., Asche, C. V., & Fairchild, C. J. (2011). The Economic Burden of Dry Eye Disease in the United States: A Decision Tree Analysis. *Cornea, 30*(4), 379–387. https://doi.org/10.1097/ico.0b013e3181f7f363.

You, Y., Qu, N., & Yu, X. (2016). Alcohol consumption and dry eye syndrome: a Meta-analysis. *International Journal of Ophthalmology.* https://doi.org/10.18240/ijo.2016.10.20.

REFERRAL WEBSITE FOR MY FAVORITE OMEGA-3 SUPPLEMENT

(I would get a small commission at no additional cost to you):

The DE3 formula (3 capsules per day) or DE Omega benefits in liquid formula (1 tsp per day). They also have other formulas for kids and if you have macular degeneration. Yes, they may seem more expensive, but when you compare the amount of omega-3s per dose and the efficacy of treating dry eyes, they are the same or more economical than most other omega-3s on the market. Make sure you compare apples to apples (the number of omega-3s per dose per dollar cost). I have one patient with HSV keratitis and dry eye disease only in one eye who called the PRN-brand fish oil "magic fish pills" as they make his eyes feel normal.

Nutriceutical Eye Supplements - Doctor Recommended | PRN. (2019, February 1). Physician-Recommended Nutriceuticals.

https://bit.ly/44cB7px

ABOUT THE AUTHOR

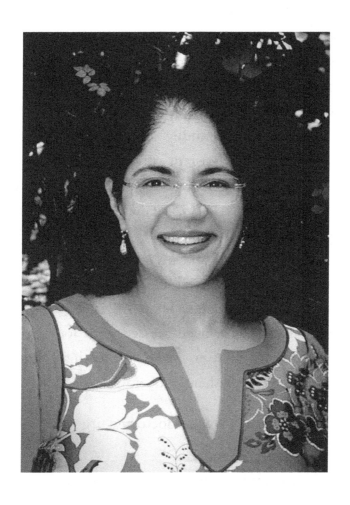

I, Dr. Shilpi Pradhan, MD, am a board-certified Ophthalmologist. I went to college at Emory University in Atlanta, GA, and medical school at Washington University in St. Louis, School of Medicine in St. Louis, MO, graduating in 2004, almost twenty years ago. I completed my one-year transitional or general medicine and surgery internship at the Carilion Clinic in Roanoke, VA, my three-year Ophthalmology residency training at the Medical College of Virginia (MCV) with Virginia Commonwealth University (VCU) in Richmond, Virginia, and my one-year Cornea and External Diseases Fellowship at the University of Pittsburgh Medical Center (UPMC) in Pittsburgh, PA. I have been in private practice since training at many private practices, including being an assistant professor at Saint Louis University in St. Louis, MO, in 2012. I opened my practice, Eye Doctor MD PC, in 2015 in Glen Allen, VA. I became a dry eye specialist because of my dry eye disease and looking for solutions for myself and my patients. I became board-certified in Lifestyle Medicine in 2020 to expand my nutrition and health knowledge. I am married to Dr. Kumar Abhishek, and we have been blessed with four children. I have helped my children self-publish their stories on Amazon as well. Check them out below:

My Website: https://www.eyedoctormd.org/

My YouTube channel: https://www.youtube.com/@ drshilpipradhan

ALSO BY SHILPI PRADHAN, MD

I've helped my children write and publish books. Please check them out below. If you love them, please leave a <u>5-star rating on Amazon, and write a review on Amazon</u> to help spread joy, cheer, and knowledge. We appreciate it!

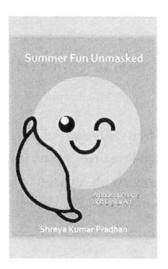

Summer Fun Unmasked: This is a book of poems and stories written by my oldest child, Shreya Kumar Pradhan, during her 4th grade virtual year at home and illustrated during the pandemic summer of 2021, published in the summer of 2021.

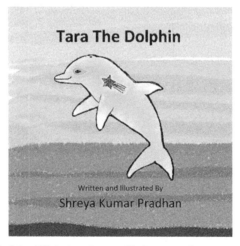

Tara the Dolphin: This is a beautiful story about a magical dolphin who teaches kindness through her magic. Written, Illustrated, and published in the spring of 2022 by my daughter, Shreya Kumar Pradhan. This story has inspired many other children to start writing their own stories.

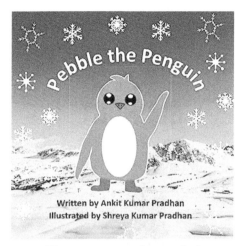

Pebble the Penguin: This is a story about a baby penguin who loves to tell jokes, written by my son who also loves to tell jokes and illustrated in a hybrid format using photos for the backgrounds from Pexels and drawings by my daughter. Published in the fall of 2022—written by my son, Ankit Kumar Pradhan, and illustrated by Shreya Kumar Pradhan.

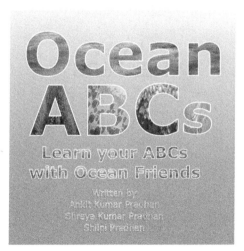

Ocean ABCs: This is a photo book about ocean animals to learn your ABCs and fun facts about ocean friends written by my oldest two kids and myself as a joint fun project, published in the winter of 2022. Written by Ankit, Shreya, and myself. Photos from free images on Pexels or Pixabay.

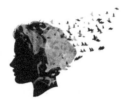

THRIVING
— **AFTER** —
BURNOUT

A Compilation of Real Stories
By Female Physicians

Guided By Sharon T McLaughlin MD FACS

I also have a chapter in the book Thriving After Burnout about my story overcoming burnout, published in January of 2023.

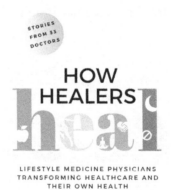

STORIES
FROM 33
DOCTORS

**HOW
HEALERS**
heal

LIFESTYLE MEDICINE PHYSICIANS
TRANSFORMING HEALTHCARE AND
THEIR OWN HEALTH

COMPILED BY:
SHILPI PRADHAN, MD

I also have a pending book coming out in July 2023 called How Healers Heal, which shares stories of transformation from 33 physicians, all board certified in Lifestyle Medicine. Be sure to check out that book as well as my chapter on fertility in that book.

www.HowHealersHeal.com

Made in the USA
Monee, IL
05 January 2024

51228123R00069